A Woman's Book of Yoga

A Woman's

MACHELLE SEIBEL, M.D., *and* HARI KAUR KHALSA

PHOTOGRAPHY BY RALPH MERCER

Avery
a member of
Penguin Putnam Inc.
New York

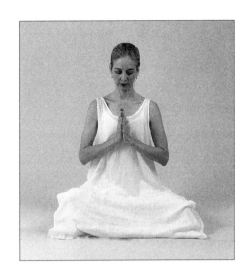

Book of Yoga

Embracing

Our Natural

Life Cycles

a member of
Penguin Putnam Inc.
375 Hudson Street
New York, NY 10014
www.penguinputnam.com

Copyright © 2002 by Machelle Seibel, M.D., and Hari Kaur Khalsa
Foreword, kriyas, meditations, and quotations copyright © 1969–2002 Yogi Bhajan
All rights reserved. This book, or parts thereof, may not be reproduced in any form without permission.
Published simultaneously in Canada

Mind-Body Connection of Reproduction diagram on page 75 copyright © 1993 Consumers Union of U.S. Inc., Yonkers, NY 10703, a nonprofit organization. Reprinted with permission for educational purposes only. No commercial use or photocopying permitted. To learn more about Consumers Union, log on to www.ConsumerReports.org.

Pregnancy Weight Record table on page 129 modified from *Journal Babies*, by M. M. Seibel and J. Stephenson (Apple Tree Press, 2000). Used with permission.

Appendix A modified from *The Soy Solution for Menopause: The Estrogen Alternative*, by Machelle M. Siebel (Fireside, 2003). Used with permission.

Interior photographs by Ralph Mercer
Yoga poses demonstrated by Christine L. Fingado, Eric Gould, Melissa Johnston, Michele Laura, Shelly Loheed, and Ruthellen Perry

Library of Congress Cataloging-in-Publication Data

Seibel, Machelle M.
   A woman's book of yoga : embracing our natural life cycles / Machelle Seibel and Hari Kaur Khalsa ; photography by Ralph Mercer.
      p.   cm.
   ISBN 1-58333-137-9 (alk. paper)
      1. Yoga, Hatha.   2. Women—Health and hygiene.   3. Exercise for women.   4. Yoga.   I. Khalsa, Hari Kaur.   II. Title.
   RA781.7 .S434   2002   2002018699
   613.7'046—dc21

Printed in the United States of America
10   9   8   7   6   5   4   3   2   1

This book is printed on acid-free paper. ∞

Book design by Lee Fukui

Acknowledgments

This project would not have been possible had I not had the good fortune to meet Yogi Bhajan, a master of Kundalini Yoga. Through my study with him, I have personally benefited from yoga and meditation practice and the yogic lifestyle. I have also had the great honor of being in his presence. The countless women who have benefited from his teachings continue to be inspired by and grateful for his tireless energy and limitless love and respect for women and all humankind.

I also dedicate this work to my mother, Gloria. She is truly a saintly woman: strong, patient, kind, compassionate, and noble. I am grateful to have had Gloria as a role model.

This book is the result of my friendship with Dr. Machelle Seibel, whose commitment to healing women reached far beyond his medical office. After attending my Kundalini Yoga classes and experiencing the benefits of yoga, meditation, and relaxation, Dr. Seibel was eager to incorporate these practices into his holistic approach to medicine. I believe this is truly a breakthrough project: a Western medical doctor working directly with a yogini to bring the best of both worlds together for the benefit of all women. Mache is a yogin, a healer, a scientist, and an artist. On behalf of myself, my yoga community, and all who will benefit from *A Woman's Book of Yoga,* we extend our gratitude for the gift of your courage, your dedication to health and healing, and your compassion.

I am grateful to Gurucharan Singh Khalsa, my first yoga teacher, for his integrity in spreading these teachings so I could grow and become a teacher myself. We share a vision of light.

I also wish to thank, from the bottom of my heart, all my fellow yoga teachers. Thank you for your ongoing support as we continue to reach out to serve and help all those in need.

Thank you to my many wonderful students for their commitment and dedication to yoga. They are a constant source of inspiration.

Thank you to my husband, Dave, who has supported my work on every level. *A Woman's Book of Yoga* could not have been completed without his help and personal support. I have a true yogic marriage—two bodies, one soul. Thank you, Dave, for your creativity, guidance, spirit, love, . . . everything.

I also want to thank Katherine Roberts, a new yoga student, who helped with the preparation of the manuscript. Her input was invaluable, and I am grateful for her assistance.

Special thanks to: KRI, Irene Frank, Gilda Forte, Hari Charn Kaur Khalsa, Hari Simran Kaur Khalsa, Shanti Shanti Kaur Khalsa, Nam Kaur Khalsa, Peg Dowd and Janet Bonner, Gina Cronin, Ron Ponte, and Bill Graham for intelligent support on every level—you are an excellent teacher, Ralph Mercer, Satya Kaur Khalsa, Manjit Kaur Khalsa, Jacob Braverman, Pat Hansen for ayurvedic healing recipes and advice, Dr. Kartar Singh Khalsa and his cleansing program, and Linda Chapman for providing the beautiful handmade yoga clothing for the models. And my appreciation to the models: Christine L. Fingado, Eric Gould, Melissa Johnston, Michele Laura, Shelly Loheed, and Ruthellen Perry.

Hari Kaur Khalsa

Long ago I realized that medicine was changing. The primary goal of medicine is no longer curing disease but helping people prevent it. When diseases and illnesses eventually do occur, it is the doctor's mission not only to assist in the healing process but also to provide support and guidance while the patient mends. I wish to thank my patients for helping to teach me these lessons. I am also indebted to Hari Kaur Khalsa, my coauthor, for providing a magnificent role model for spiritual healing—a healing art without which physical healing is incomplete. Thank you also to my wife, Sharon, and my children, Amy, Sherry, and Alex, for their support and love during the compilation of this book. I could not have completed it without their help and understanding.

Machelle M. Seibel, M.D.

Contents

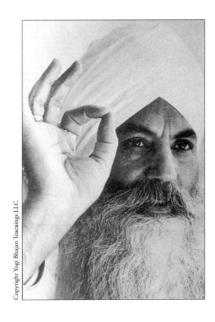

Foreword

A human being has three aspects: soul, mind, and body. When mind, body, and soul are under your control and in balance, you have gem-quality behavior, which is priceless. It makes you elegant; it makes you attractive; it gives you sacredness; it gives you respect; and it gives you wisdom. Every faculty that you need comes to you from the combination of these three.

The Sikh scriptures say woman is the source of consciousness. You play a fundamental human role in uplifting the consciousness of humanity. If humanity has been sustained up until today, it is because of the temperamental tolerance of woman. Your learning, love, and nobility can enter into the bloodstream of the generations that will follow you, bringing grace and dignity to the place where you live, and it can build a new nation and a new time.

Yogi Bhajan
Siri Singh Sahib of the Ministry of Sikh Dharma
   in the Western Hemisphere
Master of Kundalini Yoga
Founder, 3HO Foundation

Preface

Women are the embodiment of creative energy. Intuitively we know this. When we see a pregnant woman, we see the miracle even though a baby is born every minute. When we see a woman relaxed, empowered, and self-assured, the power is evident. Kundalini Yoga can bring to each woman a deep sense of her original royalty, nobility, health, happiness, and identity. The journey of the yogini—the female yogi—is one that leads through the science of learning about the body, through the revelation of the mind and its nature and capacities for bliss, and the expansiveness of the experience of the soul. This journey can lead to an acceptance and love of the self that reveals the natural radiance that is the birthright of every woman.

Women thrive from practicing this science and art of self-illumination. Unfortunately, modern culture does not uplift the feminine spirit, so young women have difficulty finding role models to help guide them toward finding their health and radiance. Women struggle to compete with one another and are deflated by the media's pervasive negative images of them.

Despite all of this, women can and do lift themselves up, find their power, and teach their daughters how to grow into self-assured women. Both the modern science of the body and the philosophy and practice of Kundalini Yoga can help all women—young and old—find the way. Understanding the basic scientific facts of a woman's physiology can enable women to take informed and positive care of their bodies. The teachings of Kundalini Yoga are powerful and timeless. They can point you in a positive direction and help you improve your mental, physical, and spiritual health. The meditations presented here are effective and can bring about real and lasting transformation.

Yogi Bhajan brought these teachings of Kundalini Yoga to the women in the United States from the East in the late 1960s. Throughout his life, he has witnessed the effects of society's degradation of women and, as a result, has dedicated his life to raise the status of women from "chicks" to eagles.

We have written this book to reach all women of all ages. When the science of the body becomes an expression of the soul, medicine and yoga have merged. It is our hope that as you read through this book, meditate on the quotes and questions, learn about your body, and discover yourself, you will be inspired to practice, teach, and enjoy each breath living in the light of your own radiance.

Hari Kaur Khalsa
Machelle Seibel, M.D.

Yoga for You

Kundalini Yoga will teach you the secret of how to be Healthy, Happy, and Holy. Kundalini Yoga will make out of you a complete, happy human being. It will develop your undeveloped corners. It will give you Grace at the weakest points of your life. It will give you what you have thought not to achieve. Kundalini Yoga is the science of living as a complete woman.

—YOGI BHAJAN

Yoga is for everyone. Yoga is for you. You can begin your yoga practice at any age, in any physical condition, and in any place where you can take a deep breath. For women, the benefits of yoga are vast, limited only by the amount of time and the degree of commitment that a person brings to it. Even for the busiest women, a few minutes of yoga practice each day can bring benefits. Moreover, it can be easily integrated into your daily schedule. You can enroll in a yoga class and benefit from the power of group practice and the social aspect of classes, or you can do yoga wherever you are at home: while the kids are napping, while nursing your baby, or in a hotel room on a business trip.

Most women who practice yoga do not have years of technical training or extraordinary flexibility. What women who practice yoga—yoginis—do have are the tools for accessing the depth and reality of their inner selves. Through the physical and mental practices of yoga, a woman can achieve deep relaxation that helps maintain inner peace and a positive self-image.

Yoga is especially helpful for the natural transitions of life. In this book, you will find many simple practices to help you stay healthy, calm, and strong, and to carry you forward in a natural progression toward wisdom, real beauty, and the strength of realized grace that belongs to all women.

This book is divided into sections so you can readily choose the specific aspects of yoga practice that most apply to your individual situations and needs. Here is what you will find in the book:

- How to use breathing, postural, and meditation exercises to optimize your health and how to adapt them to fit into busy schedules. (We will suggest both minimum and ideal amounts of time for the different exercises.)

- Specific sections and activities for general female health, menstruation, pregnancy and childbirth, perimenopause and menopause, natural beauty, and self-healing.

- Explanations of yoga exercises and meditations, each accompanied by their benefits.

- The science of stress and how yoga can help relieve stress.

- The scientific basis for the beneficial effects of yoga.

- How to determine and enhance, according to ancient wisdom, your own unique female relationship with your body, mind, and soul, and the cycles you experience.

- How to use yoga for improved sexuality and intimacy.

- How, from the yoga perspective, to improve nutrition and digestion, vital factors for good health.

This book's unique female orientation comes from the rich tradition of Kundalini Yoga. *Kundalini* means "the curl of the lock of hair of the beloved," a metaphor to describe the presence of universal energy and consciousness within each one of us. The kundalini energy is feminine in nature and is often referred to as *Mata Shakti*, the feminine Mother energy of creation. The practices described here enhance the process of merging our individual awareness with this universal Self within—how we can uncoil and awaken that feminine energy and integrate it into our lives. While yoga is essentially a spiritual path, it is at the same time a process that contributes to better physical, mental, and emotional health. Some practitioners seek the spiritual benefits. Others seek the relaxation and stress relief it brings. Others practice it for specific health benefits. The choice is yours.

In the Indian tradition, the merging of individual consciousness with universal consciousness is said to create a "divine union." In ancient Sanskrit, the word for "union" is *yoga*. In this sense, Kundalini Yoga is totally universal and nondenominational, and the students who practice it represent all religions, races, and ethnic groups.

In the chapters to follow, you will encounter much new information that, at first, may seem a bit overwhelming. Although the technical details of all aspects of yoga practice seem complex, they all come together naturally and easily in an actual practice session. Assimilate the technical information in *A Woman's Book of Yoga* as best as you can but focus on developing a simple practice. Don't be concerned if all the subtleties and aspects of yoga are not clear to you at first. Yoga practice is in the **experience**, not in the intellectual knowledge gained along the way. Use the "Yoga at Home" guides at the end of each chapter to help you simplify your approach, and take your time absorbing the depth of the Kundalini Yoga tradition.

In this chapter, we will concentrate on some of the primary aspects that make up the rich tradition of Kundalini Yoga.

Yoga, Energy, and Your Subtle Anatomy

There are "invisible" parts of yourself which are called your *Subtle Anatomy* in yoga. Just as your physical body is made up of complex layers, so is your Subtle Anatomy, but because of its elusive nature, it may be harder to understand and appreciate. The "invisible" parts of you can be defined in several ways: as your chakras, the Ten Bodies, the meridians (channels through which your energy flows), your prana and apana (generating and eliminating energies), your Moon Centers, and the kundalini energy.

For the purposes of this book, we are going to emphasize the essential concepts of Subtle Anatomy that form the basis of achieving the goal of yoga, synchronization, and the Still Point. We also devote an entire chapter of this book to the Moon Centers, which are unique to women. Knowledge of the Moon Centers can build awareness and effectiveness in a woman's life.

When we speak of "energy" in yoga, we are referring to the energy of your body and mind. Physically, energy is the movement you have in a particular physiological system—your circulatory, nervous, or glandular system. The energy of your Subtle Self becomes evident when you direct your awareness or attention toward a certain end, either to move a part of your body or to manifest a new idea. Energy and movement follow your intention or thought. Your thoughts, intentions, and the focus of your awareness are vital because they signal a chain of events that can ultimately end in an action or manifestation of word or deed. Kundalini Yoga is the art of stimulating, accessing, and directing your energy.

There are two major types of energy flows in your body: prana and apana. *Prana* is the generating energy located in the upper body, chest, heart, and rib cage. *Apana* is the eliminative energy located below the diaphragm and has a natural downward flow. During your yoga practice, the exercises, breathing techniques, meditations, and especially the Root Lock (discussed in Chapter 2) all help you direct your energy.

Prana and apana mix together in the area of your belly called your navel point. As these energies mix, the resulting downward pressure stimulates the upward flow of kundalini energy. The kundalini energy uncoils and then rises, bringing you a new level of increased sensitivity and awareness. The rising of kundalini energy is a natural response to yoga practice and to events in life that deeply inspire you (like seeing the birth of your child or reading a passage of text or scripture that you connect with). Kundalini energy is considered the energy of the soul. When you experience this energy you feel awakened, sensitive, and aware of your potential; when you directly experience your expansive nature and limitless mind, while still feeling grounded and relaxed, you are in touch with the Mother energy of kundalini.

Your Subtle Anatomy can be vital, radiant, and effective, despite the physical condition of your body. Many elderly masters can teach powerfully, despite illnesses and infirmities. This is because they can master the use of all their spiritual bodies, beyond the physical. They can perceive by using their subtlety, and they know their minds. Their pranic body serves them through their breath and energizes all other bodies. They have the capability of communicating from their chakras to your chakras, beyond the intellect, so you understand them, and their words reach your heart.

This ability to live in both the physical and subtle realms is your capacity as a woman. As you increase your knowledge of both your physical and Subtle Anatomy, you can better understand aging, cope with physical challenges and pain, and project truth and light through the most chaotic situations. Navigating your life with an understanding of your subtlety brings grace. This grace can guide you through your transitions with a broader understanding of their deeper meaning.

The many detailed writings on the Subtle Anatomy, both ancient and modern, offer more information, if you choose to read further. However, the intellectual knowledge of this concept is less important than your experience, which is your best teacher. Through the process of practicing the yoga kriyas, meditations, and relaxation, you can realize the depth of subtle experience. You are already living through your Subtle Anatomy; yoga is simply naming what is already so.

The Chakras

Think of yourself as a multifaceted crystal sitting on the planet. When the light from the sun, the source of life, shines on you, you become like a prism. The light becomes refracted into a rainbow of colors that reflect the different qualities of your energy body. The light is most dense at the base of your spine, closest to the earth, and least dense at the top of your head, closest to the heavens. Where this light pools in specific densities is where your chakras, or energy centers, are located.

Each chakra is associated with a specific quality. For instance, the first chakra, closest to the earth, is related to your ability to feel grounded and secure in your life. The chakras tend to be associated with organs and glands but function independently of them as well. These pools of energy can, just as the systems in your physical body, be in balance or out of balance. The sequences of exercises in the Kundalini Yoga kriyas are designed to balance all the chakras and uncoil the kundalini energy in a gradual and balanced manner. This is one reason we do not change the order of the exercises in the kriyas, or perform any techniques for longer than recommended. The yoga is working on a subtle level as well as on the level of your physical body.

THE CHAKRAS

1. The base of your spine and anus—stability, grounding, the element of earth

2. Between your hips, including your sexual organs—creativity, sexuality, the element of water

3. Your belly or navel point, including your solar plexus—will, discipline, the element of fire

4. Your chest area, including your heart and lungs—compassion and love, the element of air

5. Your throat area, including your thyroid gland—manifesting ideas and the power of your word, the element of ether

6. Your brow point, an area in your forehead between your eyes and above your nose, including your pituitary gland—intuitive wisdom, the element of light

7. The crown of your head at the fontanel, including your pineal gland—union with cosmic energy, the element of sound

8. The area extending approximately 3–6 feet from your body, called your aura or electromagnetic field—your shield of positive energy and your radiant presence

---

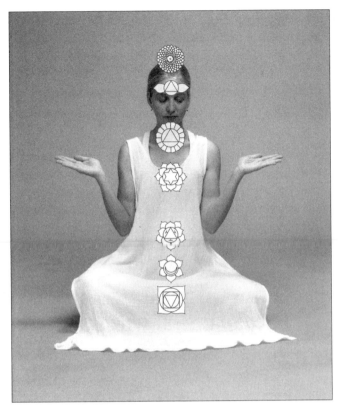

The chakras

The Ten Bodies

In addition to your chakras, you have Ten Bodies. The Ten Bodies are a further refinement of the way in which your energy manifests on the physical plane. Your Ten Bodies include your soul body, three minds (negative, positive, and neutral), physical body, arc line, aura, pranic body, subtle body, and radiant body. All of these energy bodies have unique qualities. Your soul body is timeless. Your mind is made up of three basic areas: positive, negative, and neutral (or yogic) mind. Your aura surrounds you as both a shield and a projection of energy. Your subtle body gives you the ability to perceive on a subtle level, and your radiant body is your nonlocal body, allowing you to sense things beyond the material and temporal limits of time and space.

The arc line is of special importance to women, and it is located as an arc

THE TEN BODIES

1. **Soul body**—your essence, everlasting and beyond time and space

2. **Positive mind**—collects information and analyzes how you can use it to move your projects forward, to accomplish your goals, and to be optimistic

3. **Negative mind**—helps you see what you need to avoid in order to move forward

4. **Neutral mind**—the jewel of the mind, the yoga mind, which lives a "mutual life" and has relationship without attachment—your mind working in a balanced way to see reality and experience win-win negotiations

5. **Physical body**—the temple of your spirit

6. **Arc line**—your integrity manifested in your energy, like your halo, which holds the imprint of your past actions and on which your destiny is said to be "written" and visible to those who can perceive it

7. **Aura**—your projection of light and energy, which changes subtly with each thought vibration, action, and feeling

8. **Pranic body**—the circulatory system of your Ten Bodies and your chakras, your energy level, which allows you to receive energy from the universe and to transform it into more subtle vibrations, thoughts, actions, and creativity

9. **Subtle body**—surrounds your soul and enables you to perceive detail and other aspects in the subtlest realms

10. **Radiant body**—your nonlocal experience, which enables you to sense what is happening far away as well as within range of your hearing, sight, smell, and touch—the expansiveness you feel when you have a strong ability to travel in mind and sensation beyond time and space

of light from ear to ear, like a halo. Women have an additional arc line across the chest, from one breast nipple to the other, over the heart and rib cage. These two arc lines give women additional sensitivity and radiance. The arc line represents your integrity and holds the imprint of your destiny. The pranic body is the subtle circulatory system, or connector, of all the other bodies, circulating energy throughout both your physical and Subtle Anatomy.

The Ten Bodies and Chakras

The Ten Bodies and chakras are your reality. As you practice yoga, meditation, and the breathing techniques, you can develop your ability to experience your Subtle Anatomy. This book will guide and assist you in this process. You know your physical body, and, as a woman, you know your intuition. You are more than your physical body; you are, in

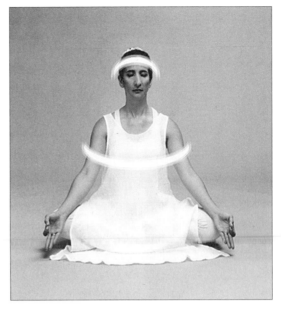

The arc lines

fact, many bodies. If your physical body is not well, then as a yogini you have other bodies to call on for support.

Synchronization—The Goal of Yoga

The goal of yoga is to reveal the connection between the human being and the Divine Self. This Divine Self, also known as God, Love, Higher Power, Universal Energy, and the Infinite, is already in all of us. The practice of yoga is a powerful way to experience this ever-present dimension. Awareness of this higher dimension of living is the basis of a sense of well-being, happiness, and healing. Ongoing experience of this dimension helps you know yourself and find your true identity. By knowing your true identity, you will experience self-love. Self-love leads to self-respect and then to the ability to be content. The ability to feel self-love and be content despite outer circumstances indicates a state of heightened awareness. Kundalini Yoga brings you to this awareness through the process of *synchronization.*

In the course of daily life, you may feel as if you are being pulled in a million directions, thinking one thing, speaking another, and juggling several tasks simultaneously without paying much attention to any one. As a result, you may feel fragmented, unfocused and stressed. When you practice Kundalini Yoga, you reverse this tendency to become fragmented by synchronizing your breathing, your physical ability to move through rhythmic exercises, and your mind (through repetition of mantra and primal sounds). The techniques of Kundalini Yoga bring body, mind, and breath into rhythmic unity. In this state of oneness is where healing can occur. The sensations of connectedness to the world and the rhythmic alignment of breath, body, and mind gained through yoga practice bring deep relief from stress and feelings of isolation and result in a sense of true relaxation.

Deep relaxation is of vital importance for women. The ancient teachings of yoga describe the female psyche as constantly operating on six levels (while men generally operate on one). The process of synchronization and core relaxation reaches all the levels of the feminine psyche and enables a woman to effectively deal with all types of stress.

The Still Point

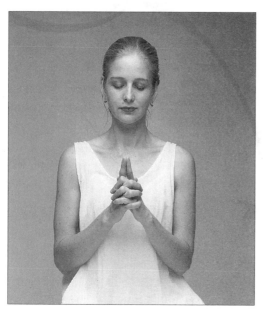

Meditative pose—the Still Point

Another basic concept in the practice of Kundalini Yoga is the Still Point. After each exercise and meditation, you will be instructed to become still, take a breath, and suspend that breath briefly, while concentrating in a particular way. The process of rhythmic movement and repeated mantra followed by concentrated stillness results in a heightened state of awareness. In this state, you can experience a stillness of both mind and body. You will experience the healing state of oneness between your finite and your Divine Self. This meditative state is the goal of yoga.

Yoga, Spirituality, and the Brain

Yoga clearly benefits the body. Practitioners of yoga are also able to experience a meditative state of mind that creates a sense of timelessness and enlightenment or, in a sense, spirituality. But how? We know intuitively that the brain creates all that we see, hear, feel, and think. Scientists in the '50s and '60s demonstrated that meditation caused changes in brainwave activity. But until recently, there was little scientific explanation for yoga's effects on the brain.

That is rapidly changing. Scientists have developed a new area of study called *neurotheology*—the study of the neurobiology of religion and spirituality. By studying yogis, Zen Buddhists, Franciscan nuns, and other deeply devout individuals of all faiths, scientists have gained a clearer understanding of the relationship between yoga and the brain.

The brain actually has a spirituality circuit that yoga and other forms of spirituality alter to ". . . create a reality different from and higher than the reality of everyday experience," according to psychologist David Wulff of Wheaton College in Massachusetts. It is a highly specialized and focused form of concentration that leads to a sense of timelessness and infinity.

To study this experience, Dr. Andrew Newberg of the University of Pennsylvania and his late colleague Dr. Eugene d'Aquili performed SPECT (single

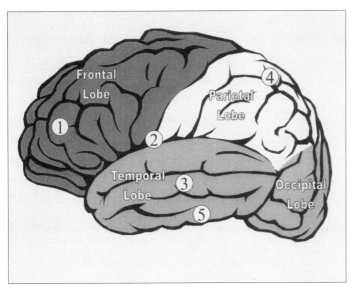

1. The frontal lobe is linked to concentration and attention. **2.** The juncture of the frontal, temporal, and parietal lobes is responsible for language, respones to religious words, and reaction to language. **3.** The middle temporal lobe contains the *amygdala* and the *hippocampus,* which together make up the *limbic* system and is involved in the emotional aspects of religion such as joy and awe. **4.** Quieting down the parietal lobes allows a person to feel at one with the universe. **5.** The lower temporal lobe facilitates prayer and meditation when exposed to images such as a cross or a Torah. (Modified from *Newsweek*, 7 May, 2001, p. 57.)

photon emission computed tomography) scans on individuals experiencing a deeply meditative state. The results were striking. The researchers were not surprised to see high activity in the prefrontal cortex, the area of the brain responsible for attention. These subjects were concentrating intently. What was surprising was the nearly total lack of activity in the superior parietal lobe, an area of the brain toward the top and back that is responsible for orienting the body in time and space. As Sharon Begley wrote in a *Newsweek* article, "Religion and the Brain," this part of the brain determines where the body ends and the rest of the world begins. The left orientation area allows us to determine where we end; the right orientation area clues us in to where we are relative to the space we occupy.

Yoga and other forms of deep meditation prevent input from getting through by creating roadblocks to these important areas of the brain. When this occurs, the brain cannot tell where the individual ends and the rest of the world begins, which creates a sense of oneness with the universe, of being in touch with infinity. According to Dr. Newberg, these experiences are not wishful thinking; they are real, biologically based events in the brain.

Studies on the *temporal lobe*, an area located on the side of the brain, have provided additional information. The temporal lobe is responsible for, among other things, the emotional aspects of religious experience, such as joy and awe (middle temporal lobe), and the process by which images such as the Torah or crosses facilitate prayer and meditation (lower temporal lobe). The middle temporal lobe contains the *amygdala* and the *hippocampus*, which together make up part of the *limbic* system, the part of the brain that deals with emotions and where memory and learning take place.

The middle temporal lobe is highly connected both to the regions of the brain responsible for motor activity and to the autonomic nervous system. Increased activity in the middle temporal lobe can therefore affect blood pressure, heart rate, and respiration (breathing). The middle temporal lobe is also directly connected to the hypothalamus, the region of the brain involved in the regulation, production, and secretion of reproductive hormones. In studies conducted by myself and Dr. Andrew Herzog of Harvard Medical School, electrical activity in the temporal lobes correlated with changes in luteinizing hormone (LH) and follicle-stimulating hormone (FSH), the two brain hormones most responsible for egg development and reproduction.

Dr. Michael Persinger of Laurentian University in Canada set out to find

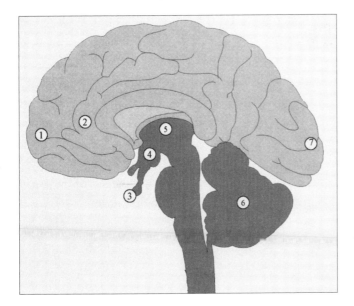

Cut section of brain (light gray) and brainstem (dark gray). **1.** The *frontal lobe* is the point of higher thought. Aging is associated with shrinkage in this area and loss of attention span. **2.** The *anterior cingulate gyrus* is responsible for impulse control and helps regulate emotions. **3.** The *pituitary gland* releases the hormones of reproduction, thyroid, and adrenal gland regulation. It is largely under the control of **4.** the *hypothalamus* and **5.** the *thalamus*. **6.** The *cerebellum* controls balance and coordination. **7.** The *visual cortex* interprets the images seen by our eyes. It is the eye and not the visual cortex that weakens with age, making seeing more difficult. The hippocampus, hidden below and behind the thalamus, is essential for forming and retrieving memories and may account for those senior moments. (Modified from *Newsweek*, Special Issue Fall/Winter 2001, pp. 28–29.)

whether short bursts of electrical activity in one or both temporal lobes could create spiritual experiences. Volunteers were asked to wear a helmet containing electromagnets that created a weak magnetic field in the temporal lobes. What they described were spiritual and out-of-body experiences that created a sense of the divine. The conclusion was that stimulating the left temporal lobe, which maintains our sense of self, while keeping the right temporal lobe quiet causes the brain to perceive a presence or the self departing the body, or even the presence of God. These experiences are not isolated events or the exclusive results of fancy scientific experiments but can occur naturally. In fact, Gallup polls in the '90s found that more than half of American adults have experienced "a moment of sudden religious awakening or insight."

Others, such as psychologist Richard Bentall of the University of Manchester in England, have studied Broca's area of the brain, the part responsible for speech. He believes that hearing the voice of God, or our higher Divine Self, could in reality be the inner voice of our own thoughts caused by Broca's area switching on at the same time that meditation or prayer is dampening sensory input. The end result is a sense that the inner voice is coming from an external source, such as the voice of God.

Yoga may contribute to a sense of spirituality in other ways as well. Studies have shown that rituals, such as drumming, dancing, and incantations, that cause us to focus intently can also evoke intense emotions—one of yoga's objectives. Through a combination of body movements (exercises), mantras (sounds), repetitive breathing (breath of fire and other breathing techniques), and concentration (focus on our brow point, sound, or hand/body pose), yoga combines the elements necessary to open the door to spirituality and oneness.

How? By tuning out the extraneous sensory stimuli and activating the temporal lobe, the intense focus leads to heightened emotions. An intense focus also decreases input from the hippocampus to the orientation area of the parietal lobe, the area that tells us where our self ends and the rest of the world begins. Add to this an activation of the parasympathetic nervous system and you have an explanation of how yoga helps to achieve relaxation and a heightened sense of spirituality.

The Foundation of Yoga Techniques

When you build a house, you need a solid foundation. When you work with raising the energy of awareness in your body in order to connect with your Divine Self and the potential within, you work from the foundation of your beliefs and values, on which your attitudes and actions are based. As you practice yoga, you begin to feel empowered, positive, and energized in mind and body. Your basic values and disciplines determine how you will manifest this energy in the world. Yoga has a philosophical model that helps you direct your energy toward both your own higher good and the good of the world. This model is an eight-stage path toward purification of the mind:

1. *Yama*—The values you hold for how you interact with your world: nonhurting, nonlying, nonstealing, nonpossessive (nongreed).

2. *Niyama*—The values you hold for how you treat yourself: purity, contentment, purification, and zeal (for your practice and study); study, devotion, and surrender (allowing yourself to feel expansive).

3. *Asana*—The practice of postures for health that prepare you to relax enough to meditate. "How you hold yourself, who you are. What you are. How flexible and rigid you are" (Yogi Bhajan).

4. **Pranayama**—The managing and directing of your energy or life force, often through breathing techniques. "How expanded, powerful, energetic you are" (Yogi Bhajan).

5. **Pratyahar**—The synchronization of your senses and thoughts. Pratyahar is also considered the state of sense withdrawal, the time in meditation when your brainwave activity shifts and your senses no longer distract you from the act of meditation. "How humble and synchronized you can be" (Yogi Bhajan).

6. **Dharana**—Attaining one-pointed concentration. "How much you can flow into the attunement of the flow of your life" (Yogi Bhajan).

7. **Dhyana**—Deep meditation. "How meditative, concentrative, solid you are to beam and achieve" (Yogi Bhajan).

8. **Samadhi**—Awakening to and absorption in Spirit. "How blissful in ecstasy you are to be grateful" (Yogi Bhajan).

The foundation of the yogic path lies in the *yama*s and *niyama*s, which help direct your mind toward positive use of your energy. States Yogi Bhajan: "Every day wasted without Yam and Niyam, without do's and dont's, is denying a stage of ecstasy. It is based on the law of nature, Mother Nature." All eight steps help you assess your integrity, both within yourself and in your world. Have faith in your ability to create positive changes in your body and your thinking. With this first step you can develop more positive attitudes about yourself and a more relaxed approach to the world. You may be able to see your life in a larger perspective, which can point you toward living a true, healthy, happy, and integrated life.

Each practice session ideally includes exercise, meditation, relaxation, and contemplation. In this manner, you create a solid foundation as well as touch upon all the steps on the path each time you practice. Take your time. Yoga can be a powerfully transforming experience. Relax and approach your practice with common sense, patience, and a sacred attitude.

Sound, Mantra, and Your Mind

Every element of the universe, which is manifested to us as light, sound, and energy, is in a constant state of vibration. Your senses perceive only a fraction of the infinite range of this vibration. You can tune your mind into the awareness of that totality with the use of sound and mantra. By vibrating, by chanting in rhythm with your breath using a particular sound, you can expand your sensitivity to the entire spectrum of vibrations. It is similar to striking a note on a stringed piano. As you vibrate, the universe vibrates with you.

Your body is a divine instrument that responds to both the outer vibrations and impressions of your environment and to your inner thought vibrations. Through yoga you learn to play this instrument in tune with the Divine Self, or Divine Vibration—the pulse of life. You use your own vibration and sound as a powerful healing tool.

The science of yoga acknowledges the powerful impact of both the vocal and silent vibrations of your word. Your thoughts are silently repeated vibrations that affect your moods. You already know how powerful your words are. Have you ever said something and wanted to "take it back"? Have you noticed the direct link between your thoughts and the way you feel or act? Your thought vibrations color how you perceive your world. Your thoughts become words, which create relationships and communicate knowledge and wisdom. In the philosophy of yoga, we go as far as saying that these mental projections actually *create* your world. How you sense, act, and react is largely in response to your thinking.

Sound and mantra are fundamental, powerful tools in the practice of Kundalini Yoga. Through the use of sound and mantra, you can attain deep meditative states that bring you to self-realization. Mantras are not ordinary words; they are special sounds, primal vibrations that align with the frequency of the vibration of your Divine Self.

From a physical perspective, the roof of your mouth has eighty-four meridian points, similar to the energy channels used in acupuncture. Each time you make a sound, your tongue stimulates the eighty-four subtle meridian points on the roof of your mouth. Stimulating these points in various combinations has a direct impact on your brain and helps to create the hormonal and chemical changes indicative of meditative states and states of deep relaxation.

The repetition of mantras, called *jaapa,* is a fast, effective practice that focuses your mind and changes the pattern of distracting thoughts by replacing them with vibrations that stimulate awareness and your highest potential. Jaapa has the power to break deeply held, unhealthy patterns in your temperament and has a healing effect on your mind. Using mantras also results in mind/body synchronization, thus creating the Still Point, as you repeat them while doing physical exercise, breathing techniques, and meditations.

Yoga and the Body

As you practice yoga, you begin to pay attention to the sensations you feel in your body. Take a moment and ask yourself how you feel about your body. Based on your past, present, and future hopes and fears, you have developed a unique relationship with your body. Your thoughts about your body—how it feels and how it looks—help create this relationship. The yogini's view of the body is simple: The body is your temple. The temple of the body is the vehicle for your soul. Your body is a complex vehicle through which you experience your life. It has a capacity for sensation, healing and regeneration, and brilliant radiance. Whatever your relationship is with your body now, whatever phase of life you are in, the practice of yoga can raise your awareness so that you have a more positive relationship with your body.

For a beginning yoga student, the first effect of yoga practice is body awareness. Increased body awareness calls attention both to the thoughts you have about your body (including your flexibility or stiffness) and to issues with your weight, strength, and vitality. Confronting these issues can be difficult. Remember that the practice of yoga is a journey of self-knowledge and that the self-knowledge you gain is the first step in accepting your present state of health. From a clear and realistic understanding of your present state of physical health, you can consciously and gradually move toward healing and increased energy to meet the challenges of life.

As you practice yoga exercises in this book, remember to appreciate your body as it is, to practice self-acceptance, and to release the expectations of how your body should look. The expectations you have regarding how you look are often based on cultural stereotypes or trends. Often these trends are not realistic and do not encourage women to be healthy and happy. Cultivate a positive relationship with your body. Keep in mind these words from a song in our yoga practice: "I am who I am and that is that." The meditations and techniques presented in this book echo this thought. They can also help you cut through and eliminate the thoughts that do not empower your self-image.

Breath

You can do yoga without postures and exercises, but you cannot do yoga without conscious attention to your breath. Breath can be considered the physical counterpart of your mind. While *mind, consciousness,* and *Divine Self* are abstract terms, breath is a physical reality. Through the experience of the movement of your breath, you link your physical reality to your abstract and expanded consciousness. Through the practice of breathing techniques and the focusing of your attention on your breath, the yogini directs her prana, her vital energy, and her attention. This science of controlling and directing energy through breath practices is called *pranayama*. Kundalini Yoga includes different types of breathing techniques that have particular effects on the body and mind. As you apply your conscious attention to breathing techniques, you increase your prana. You need strong prana to penetrate negativity and maintain self-love as your primary focus. The breathing techniques are powerful and effective in accumulating this inner-core prana. At the same time, these techniques help release tension, toxins, and pain from your body.

While people practice yoga techniques, the mind has a tendency to "go shopping," or to wander (review the past or project into the future). In Kundalini Yoga, the breath is often linked to a specific sound, a *mantra*. As you repeat the mantra with each breath, you direct your prana toward a frequency that links you with higher states of consciousness. The repetition of the sound in rhythm with breath and/or body movement cuts through the distractions of the wandering, grasping, or "shopping" mind and creates the synchronization of your mind, body, and breath. The result of this synchronization is a single-pointed and relaxed state.

One of the traditional mantras used in Kundalini Yoga is *Sat Naam* (pronounced *sut nahm*). It is a *bij mantra,* a seed mantra that works at a primal subconscious level to elevate your consciousness. *Sat* means "your truth, your essence"—the very seed from which your honest words and actions grow. *Naam* means "vibration," or "identity"—the expression of your essence in the world. *Sat Naam* can be translated as "Your identity is Truth," "True Name," or "True Self." The meaning of the word *truth* in this sense refers to your experience of reality, here and now, in the present moment. With each breath, yoga can be said to join your *Sat* with your *Naam,* join your truth and reality with your identity. While other traditions use different mantras and sounds, these particular sounds produce the best results in Kundalini Yoga practice. This mantra is linked to each breath: On each inhalation you mentally chant *Sat,* and on each exhalation, *Naam.* The result of this technique is a focused mind that expresses the very essence of your true identity and destiny with each action and word.

Meditation

You are what you think. Your mental projection is the highest projection in the existence in the human body. Nothing comes from outside. —Yogi Bhajan

Meditation—the mastery of your mind—is the most important challenge for women. How we think directly affects how we feel and how we act. Meditation is the science and art of creating positive and healthy thoughts that result in actions that correspond with your highest intentions. Many meditations included in this book directly address your pituitary gland and your brain chemistry, which, in turn, affect your hormonal balance. Although we do not, at this writing, scientifically understand exactly how meditation works or why it works so well, we do know that your brain chemistry affects your moods and thoughts, and vice versa.

Your mind generates a thousand thoughts per blink of your eye. Some of those thoughts are perceived consciously, and some go into your subconscious. The millions of thoughts and impressions stored in your subconscious can interfere with your ability to focus and act with clarity. When impressions from your past, stored in your subconscious, enter into your conscious behavior without your knowledge, you begin to act out of past fears and experiences instead of present realities. The process of meditation can prevent this common tendency.

Meditation is a process that provokes your subconscious and helps to "dump out" or eliminate your unwanted fears and thought patterns. You may have many distracting thoughts as you meditate, especially during the early stages of your meditation practice. This is not uncommon and is part of the meditation experience. It is the process of eliminating those negative thoughts (or cutting through them and replacing them with thoughts of higher vibrations such as mantras) that creates mastery over the chaos of your mind and leads you toward stillness and clarity. Emptying the garbage isn't always pleasant, but it feels great when it is gone. Be patient and persistent and let the process work.

In meditation, you train your mind to be relaxed, creative, and focused. You can learn to be more responsible for your thoughts. Says Yogi Bhajan: "Every thought becomes an emotion, a feeling, a desire. It's endless. And it's like a fire. The more wood [thoughts] you put on it, the more it burns; and the more it burns, the more it needs. Desires are like that. The more you desire, the more you go after it." By creating calm and quiet through the disciplined release of mental tension, meditation can free you from the cycle of grasping outside yourself for the value and contentment that are really located within you. Meditation is thus said to break the illusion of desire on the earth plane.

With mastery over your mind, you can master your life. Meditation is especially important during your life's transitions, when your brain and body chemistry challenges you with fluctuations that result in mood swings and intense mental states. Meditation is powerful enough, when done with honesty and intention, to change your brain chemistry and bring you to a more balanced state. Meditation can shift how you perceive your body and pain. Mantra and breath meditations can be especially effective in creating positive change during these times. There are different meditation techniques from many traditions. Kundalini Yoga employs a variety of techniques using breath, mantra, sound, and visualization. In this way, the meditations you will learn in this book can balance and stimulate specific areas of your brain and synchronize your entire being.

The techniques of Kundalini Yoga are designed to help you access the powerful feminine energy within you and to bring you to a meditative state in tune with your Divine Self. The yoga itself is not the goal, but it is the key to opening the door to health, self-love, and self-realization. As you read on, you will learn how yoga automatically, gently, and widely opens this door.

Bringing the Art of Yoga and Relaxation into Your Life: Questions for Further Growth

- What times of day are you most stressed or rushed? Can you imagine taking some extra time each day to relax and pay attention to your body, mind, and spirit?

- Are there times in your life when you experience the Still Point— moments of feeling at one with the world and at peace? Yoga teaches you how to create that feeling on command. How can this be of benefit to you?

- The journey of yoga is the journey toward self-love and self-respect of your body, mind, and spirit. What is your present level of physical fitness? What are your current feelings toward your body?

- The yoga of sound and mantra will enable you to communicate consciously and will help you to create an uplifting environment for yourself. Take some time to evaluate the sounds you hear and how you speak. How do the TV, radio, and music you hear affect you? Do you have the capacity to listen as well as to communicate?

2 Preparing to Practice

Learning is not a weakness. Every process is a moment; every moment is a process. Learning is to gain wisdom. It gives us a grip on our discipline.

—YOGI BHAJAN

Before attempting to practice a complete yoga set, we recommend that you learn a few basic techniques that are essential to most sessions of Kundalini Yoga. These techniques include how to chant, breathe in a variety of ways, sit for meditation, and hold basic postures. In this chapter we will also explain various body locks, or *bhandas*—muscular contractions used to stimulate energy and align the spine—and will consider the important topics of eye focus, rhythm, and relaxation.

Take some time to familiarize yourself with each technique before moving on to your first full practice session in Chapter 3. Yoga exercises can be both gentle and rigorous. Like any other exercise program, check with your physician before beginning.

It is important before each yoga session to take a moment to create a sacred space. This sacred space will separate your yoga practice from the rest of your day and establish the best environment for personal growth.

Creating sound is both a science and an art in which you use your body as an instrument, a vibratory vessel. Before chanting either aloud or silently, follow these steps to add depth, sacredness, and impact to your experience.

1. Take a few relaxed breaths. Be aware of your breath and your environment. Listen to the sounds around you. Become sensitive to your space and thoughts—notice your internal and external environments.

2. Bring your awareness to your spine. Visualize your spinal column and, within that column, a filament pathway in the center. You are visualizing the "central channel," or *shushmana*. Now visualize the area in your forehead between your eyebrows, slightly above the top of your nose—the brow point. When you create a sound, place it in this area.

3. When you chant, listen to your own sound with total attention. As you listen, surrender your whole being to the sound you are creating. This will deepen the effects of chanting and prevent your mind from wandering.

Below is the traditional mantra vibration we use to begin a Kundalini Yoga session:

Ong Naamo

[*ong – ng nah-moh*]

Guroo Dayv Naamo

(*goo – roo* [on the *r* hit your tongue on the roof

of your mouth] *dayv nah-moh*]

This means:

I acknowledge the One Creative Consciousness

I acknowledge the Subtle and Divine Wisdom Within.

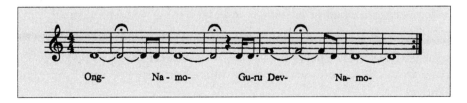

Inhale deeply and exhale as you chant *Ong Naamo*. The *ong* is long, and you vibrate the *ng* sound in your nasal cavity. Chanting the *ng* in your nasal cavity is said to stimulate your brain. Either chant the entire mantra on one breath, or take a short breath in through the mouth and exhale as you chant *Guroo Dayv Naamo*.

Repeating this mantra three or more times before each session helps you to acknowledge your connection to all and the divine wisdom within you. Starting your practice with this mantra provides the foundation for transformation and healing.

You will learn other vibrations and mantras throughout this book. Linking your breath to sound is a central aspect of Kundalini Yoga. When your breath and sound are synchronized, your yoga practice will be more powerful and effective. Master mantra and you master your mind!

How to Breathe in Yoga Practice

Diaphragmatic Breathing— Opening the Belly and Discovering the Breath

Long, Deep Breathing is the foundation of your yoga practice. This breath feeds your blood with precious oxygen, relaxes you, and heals you. The Long, Deep Breath is slow and controlled. You begin learning the Long, Deep Breath by learning diaphragmatic breathing and thus retraining your body to breathe naturally.

Begin by lying on your back and place both hands on your belly, fingers touching. Relax your belly and your chest. Inhale through your nose and feel the natural expansion of your abdomen. This lifting action will cause the fingers to separate. Exhale through your nose, completely, a slow exhale. Your abdomen will relax and your fingers will return to their original position. You will also feel the expansion of your rib cage. Try to feel this expansion as a wide opening, instead of lifting upward and tensing your shoulders. It may help to visualize your spine as a glass and your breath as light. Inhale and pour the breath, "filling the glass" from bottom up; exhale, "emptying the glass" from top to bottom. Try several times, being sure to relax your neck and jaw.

The expansion of your abdomen on your inhale indicates that you are using your diaphragm muscle, located about an inch above your belly button, to help draw breath into the lungs. You may need to exaggerate the expansion of your belly if your breath is shallow until your breath is smooth and deep, accompanied by the natural expansion of belly, lower back, and rib cage. As you begin to breathe in this natural manner, pay attention to the details of your breathing. Feel your lower back expand as you inhale. With each inhalation, your belly rises, your lower back expands out, and your rib cage expands. This will release tension from your shoulders and neck, allowing a full breath to occur and expanding your lung capacity.

Long, Deep Breathing is done primarily through your nose. Breathing through your nose warms, humidifies, and filters the air entering your lungs, so that you deliver the highest quality air to your lungs in the most efficient manner. Breathing consciously through your nose instead of your mouth will slow your breath rate, thereby facilitating higher awareness and a more relaxed state.

As you practice yoga this will become the natural way you breathe all the time. Watch any young child and you will understand how natural Long, Deep Breathing is. As we age, stress often tightens up the belly and creates the habit of breathing using the large chest muscles. Breathing correctly gives your body a precious gift. Practice Long, Deep Breathing slowly and enjoy its many benefits!

Segmented Breathing—Managing Your Moods

Segmented Breathing is a way to refine your breathing and manage your moods. Take a few long, deep breaths first, making sure you are breathing diaphragmatically. Sit straight in a chair or sit comfortably cross-legged (called Easy Pose) on a flat surface. While you are learning, you can also practice this as you lie on your back. As you inhale, break your breath into four equal segments (sniffs). Hold this breath in for a few seconds. Then exhale, breaking the breath again into four equal segments (sniffs). Hold that breath out for a few seconds. Continue inhaling in four equal segments and exhaling in four equal segments. It may take you a little while to equalize the segments and to have a complete inhale and exhale. Next, inhale in four equal segments and exhale in one long, continuous breath. Repeat this pattern a few times and feel the difference. This four/four breath, intended primarily for relaxation, is very effective in managing emotional and mental states. It also will help increase your strength, vitality, and mental focus. Segmented Breathing is a yogic gem. Once you learn it, you will have a useful tool for managing your moods.

Breath of Fire—Beating Stress

This breath technique is a super energizer and stress buster. Breath of Fire works deep in your solar plexus, located at the base of your rib cage, to engage your parasympathetic nervous system and to return it to balance, giving you strength and raising your self-esteem. Breath of Fire powerfully breaks the habit your nervous system may have developed of entering into and remaining in the stress response. Other benefits believed to come from Breath of Fire include detoxification of the blood, increased energy at the solar plexus (the third chakra, the energy center that helps energize your entire body, mind, and spirit), improved digestion, strengthened adrenal function, and enhanced mental clarity.

Breath of Fire is a rapid breath generated from the diaphragm area with a powerful but gentle pulse. Begin by lying on the floor on your back or sitting in a comfortable position. Take a few long, deep breaths. Breath of Fire is very rapid, but it is not hyperventilation. To learn how to manipulate your muscles for Breath of Fire, first inhale a slow, deep breath and suspend, or hold it without straining (see the next section). As you suspend your breath, pump your belly in and out a few times—these are the muscles you should use to breathe during this exercise. Exhale and relax. Next, stick out your tongue and pant like a dog. Just let go of your intellectualization of the process and breathe! This allows you to get the feeling of moving your navel point and using your diaphragm and abdominal muscles, both of which are necessary for Breath of Fire.

Once you are familiar with the feeling of the muscles for Breath of Fire, you may begin the practice. Sit in a comfortable position or lie on your back on the floor. Take a few long, deep breaths. Begin breathing in and out rapidly, with one sniff in for inhalation and one sniff out for the exhalation (this is similar to one segment from Segmented Breathing). Place equal emphasis on the inhalation and the exhalation, keeping your breath even and rhythmic. Your rate of breaths should be about two to three breaths per second.

Practice Breath of Fire for short periods of time, alternating with relaxed diaphragmatic breathing. With practice, you will become comfortable with Breath of Fire and energized by this technique. You should feel comfortable and relaxed while doing this breath.

Note: Breath of Fire should be practiced only very lightly during menstruation, and not at all during pregnancy and the first three months after delivery.

Suspending Your Breath—Achieving Stillness

You can affect your autonomic nervous system by consciously changing your breath rate. Changing your breath rate will bring about a shift in your physiological and mental states. Your "normal" breath rate is about twenty breaths per minute. During yoga practice, you bring the breath down to about eight breaths per minute, automatically entering a meditative state.

At the end of many exercises, you will be instructed to suspend your breath briefly before you relax. Suspending your breath is like holding your breath in or out but without the strain or tension you normally feel in your chest or shoulders. This process stimulates your experience of the Still Point (as described in Chapter 1), a basic goal of yoga and meditation.

To suspend your breath on the inhalation, inhale and retain your breath, keeping your chest expanded. If you feel any tension, let some breath out and try again. Remember to feel relaxed, even as you retain your breath. To suspend your breath on the exhalation, exhale completely, maintaining a straight spine. Whether suspending your breath in or out, relax your shoulders back and focus your eyes at your brow point. Become still and feel light and open. Hold your concentration gently at the brow in stillness. When suspending your breath after the physical experience of the exercises and the repetition of mantras, you will experience the Still Point. This stillness is in contrast to the movements just completed; it is this contrast that, in part, allows you to enter the quiet, meditative state of mind. This experience of stillness will become deeper when you apply the Root Lock, described later in this chapter.

Rhythm

Kundalini Yoga, like life itself, is rhythmic. Women naturally experience life as a rhythmic cycle, and the capacity for happiness lies in your ability to navigate through the transitions and cycles of life without resistance. In Kundalini Yoga, many meditations and exercises have an inherent rhythm. This rhythm signals your separate or dis-integrated parts to act in concert with each other. The goal of Kundalini Yoga is to integrate your finite self with infinity through rhythm. As you practice linking your breath with your movement and mantra, you will feel balanced and in harmony. When you do each exercise set in this book, start slowly. As your body becomes accustomed to moving and breathing, you can increase the speed of your movements to a steady pace.

The Art of Relaxation

Relaxation is the art of being calm in all situations. A woman's power is in her natural ability to contain her energy. A woman can naturally adjust her energy according to the needs of her life and its challenges. Although we live in a stressful world, you can learn to relax. To master relaxation is to master the flow of your life between activity and rest, between action and stillness. Remember to take time, from one to three minutes between each exercise, and from three to eleven minutes or more at the end of each practice session, to relax.

True relaxation is more than keeping your muscles still. It is a state of being in which your actions are aligned with your core beliefs and truth. Relaxation involves a sense of feeling connected to life and being at ease in the flow of your life. In order to discover your inner truth, and match your actions with it, you must gain insight into the nature of your mind and thoughts. This is why meditation is a most important part of yoga practice. The yoga exercises will create new, healthy patterns in your biological systems. The meditations will help relieve distracting thoughts and create a new template for a focused and clear mind so you can know yourself and act accordingly. By helping to integrate these new patterns into your entire being, the relaxation practice allows for real transformation.

For women, it is beneficial to relax on both the back and the belly. When you relax on your belly, you can feel the protection of Mother Earth against the front of your body—the more vulnerable part of you. Relaxing in this way can help you feel protected and secure. When you lay on your back, with your arms by your side and your palms facing up, you are open and in a position of receptivity and surrender. If you relax while in this position of openness, you can strengthen your nervous system.

To come out of a relaxation, take a few deep breaths, wiggle your toes and fingers, and rotate your wrists and ankles as you return to normal consciousness. Stretch your arms over your head and inhale. Suspend your breath briefly, and stretch and tighten all your muscles as you wake up every one of your trillions of cells. Exhale and relax. Stretch your back with a few Cat Stretches (see Chapter 10), and bring your knees to your chest and roll up and down from the base of your spine to your shoulders, to massage and stimulate your spine. Then sit up and finish your yoga set, or end your session with an affirmation of peace and healing.

Projection, Affirmation, and Prayer

End each yoga session with a moment of projection, affirmation, or prayer. From this yogic state of balance, your intentions will have added power and impact.

Mudras

*Mudra*s are hand or body postures that you hold while exercising or meditating. These positions are important because they stimulate your body, most often your nervous system, to create a certain pattern. One translation often used for the Sanskrit word *mudra* is "seal." When you hold a mudra, it "seals" a desired effect in both your body and mind. One basic and frequently mentioned hand mudra you will learn is Gyan Mudra. To do this mudra, touch your thumb to your index finger of each hand to form a circle. *Gyan* means "knowledge," and this mudra seals the quality and pattern of expansive knowledge into your body, mind, and being.

Eye Focus

Your eye focus is important during exercise, meditation, and relaxation. The major eye focus positions are as follows:

Eyes closed. Keeping your eyes closed during yoga practice, unless you need them to help you balance, is a powerful way to eliminate extra stimulation from your external environment and will encourage an inner focus.

Eyes closed and focused at your brow point. In the yogic Subtle Anatomy, this is the location of the sixth chakra or energy center, the yogic "third eye." This eye focus can help stimulate your intuition and insight.

Eyes one-tenth open or closed and focused down toward the tip of your nose. This eye focus locks your mind in a powerful concentrated focus.

Eyes closed and focused down toward the tip of your chin. This focus is used to steady your emotions.

Eyes closed and focused at the crown of your head. This focus stimulates your divine connection with infinity.

The Body Locks

The body locks are postures that are used throughout yoga practice to help you align your spine and to stimulate and direct your energy and awareness. Physically, the application of body locks changes the blood circulation, stimulates nerves, and affects the flow of spinal fluid. The practice of these locks is integral to achieving the benefits of Kundalini Yoga. Here is a brief description of three of the basic body locks.

The Root Lock—*Mula Bhandha*

Begin by sitting in Easy Pose or in a comfortable posture. To apply the Root Lock, focus on your anal sphincter, sex organs, and belly button and on your lower abdominal muscles. First, tighten the anal sphincter and then the sex organs (as if you are stopping the flow of urine), and then pull your lower belly in toward your spine. Applying the Root Lock should not feel too tense, but as if the constriction of these muscles is bringing strength and concentration to the lower muscles and chakras. When you release the Root Lock, try to sense the release of tension that relaxes your body and balances your energy. As mentioned earlier, at the end of each exercise, you can suspend your breath comfortably; focus at your brow point and apply the Root Lock briefly.

The Neck Lock—*Jalandhara Bandha*

To apply the Neck Lock, sit with your spine erect and your neck relaxed. Raise your chest slightly and pull your chin in toward your spine so the back of your neck feels elongated, but you are not strained. Stay aware of the position of your neck during yoga if a posture is a challenge for you, or if your body is not flexible, you may try to move your chin and neck more than necessary. Keep your neck relaxed and steady during yoga practice.

The Diaphragm Lock—*Uddiyana Bandha*

Locate your diaphragm muscle, then inhale deeply and exhale completely. After you exhale, hold your breath out. While holding your breath out, pull or lift the diaphragm up, as if you are bringing it up behind your ribs and into the thorax. The upper abdominal muscles are pulled in toward your spine as you lift the diaphragm. This lock is normally applied gently on the exhalation. This lock is not applied with the breath held in. This lock gives your heart a gentle massage. It also stimulates the upward flow of your energy from your belly, the third energy center, toward your heart and neck, the fourth and fifth energy centers.

How to Sit

When you practice yoga in a seated pose it is important to keep your spine erect without putting too much strain on your back. The following poses are suitable for most students.

Egyptian Pose in a Chair

Sit in a chair with your feet flat on the floor. If your feet do not reach the floor, place books or a low footstool under your feet so they are flat. Lengthen your spine and hold it away from the back of the chair. Relax your hands on your thighs.

Easy Pose

This is the most common cross-legged position. Sit on the floor and cross your legs. Your feet are tucked under the knees of the opposite leg. If you feel tension in your knees, ankles, or back, try sitting on a folded blanket or cushion. You can use the blanket or cushion each time you meditate or exercise.

Perfect Pose

Sit on the floor and bring one of your heels close into your groin. Bring your other heel to rest in the notch of the ankle of the leg closest to your groin. In this pose, your legs are not crossed; your feet are locked together at the ankle. Many people find this seated pose very comfortable.

Half-Lotus Pose

Sit on the floor in Easy Pose. Bring one of your feet up to rest on the thigh of your other leg. Allow your other foot to stay underneath. Half-Lotus provides extra support for your back by opening and locking your hips.

Full-Lotus Pose

Sit on the floor in Half-Lotus Pose. Bring the foot that is underneath your leg up through the opening between your other knee and your groin. Both feet should each be resting on the opposite thigh. This is a rigorous posture for many people. However, if your knees, hips, and ankles are flexible, you may find this the most comfortable sitting position. Full Lotus opens your hips so they can support your back.

Rock Pose

Sit on your heels on the floor. This is an excellent pose for women; it supports the back and stimulates digestion. Rock Pose puts pressure on and adjusts your reproductive organs. If you find Rock Pose comfortable, you can use it for any indicated seated exercise.

Most beginners find sitting in a chair or sitting in Easy Pose with a folded blanket or cushion to be the most comfortable sitting posture. Choose the posture that you can maintain most comfortably. Feel free to take a break and stretch out your legs whenever you need to.

A Note on Poses and Posture

Finding a comfortable posture in which to sit and meditate can be the first challenge in learning how to become still and to focus. Do not hesitate to use a chair or extra pillows so your spine can remain erect without strain. As you practice yoga, you will find that your flexibility and strength will increase and that sitting to meditate will become easier. As you actually begin to practice, all the details will begin to fit into place. Each exercise, meditation, and kriya will touch you in a new way.

It only takes a minute (less than a minute!) to take a deep breath, and conscious breathing is the beginning of training yourself to relax and bring yoga practice into your life. Ideally, yoga is practiced in the morning so you can set your mind and body for the day to come, but any time you practice you will give your mind and body a break from the stresses and routines of your day.

The First Steps to Yoga

1. Tune in with *Ong Naamo Guroo Dayv Naamo*, repeating the mantra three times or until you feel you have created a calm, sacred space. Listening is a powerful art; take a moment to relax and listen to the echoes of your vibration.

2. *Practice Long, Deep Breathing.* Use the yogic breathing system of diaphragmatic breathing, allowing the lower back and abdomen to expand as you inhale. Lie on your back for 11 minutes each day and practice this breath technique without strain or too much effort. If you have difficulty locating your breath, place a pillow on your belly and feel it lift as you inhale and come back down as you exhale. To end your practice, inhale deeply, suspend (hold) the breath briefly while you visualize energy going to all your cells, then exhale and relax. Take a few of these long, deep breaths any time you feel the need to relax and rejuvenate yourself.

3. *Root Lock.* Sitting in Easy Pose or in a comfortable seated position with your spine held straight but relaxed, inhale, apply the Root Lock, and hold for 5–10 seconds. Exhale and release the lock. Practice applying the Root Lock several times, until you can locate and tighten your pelvic floor muscles without tightening your shoulders or creating tension in other areas of your body. Do not practice the Root Lock during menstruation or pregnancy. If you are pregnant, do the Kegel exercises as described in Chapter 7.

QUESTIONS FOR FURTHER GROWTH

- How often are you in touch with your sacredness and intuition? Tuning in helps you create a sacred space that stimulates your intuition.

- What times of day are you most rushed or stressed? Can you take a few deep breaths at those times and help yourself relax and gain perspective?

- Practice the Root Lock when you need energy and to create the Still Point. How does it change your awareness?

3

A Beginning Kundalini Yoga Session

The time is now and now is the time.

—YOGI BHAJAN

The practice of yoga is designed to help you confront your negative patterns, in the interest of creating positive changes. If you do not provoke and confront your own ego, how can you transform your negativity and build new positive habits? Don't be surprised if you notice resistance to daily yoga practice or to creating any new habit in your life. The victory is in keeping your promise to yourself to make time for the self-healing and relaxation that benefit your health and well-being. Keeping this commitment to yourself is the first step toward inner happiness.

The process of transformation through yoga practice can best be described as the process of crystallization. Slowly, over time, nature pressurizes carbon until it crystallizes into a diamond. In much the same way, slowly, over time, if you apply disciplined pressure to yourself by practicing exercises, postures, and meditations, you, too, become a diamond—with a clarity that reflects the universe!

The process of "crystallization" has three stages. The first stage is called *Sadhana* (pronounced *sah-duh-nah*). The word *Sadhana* actually means "practice" or "discipline." The first step in using yoga to transform yourself, help heal an imbalance, or shift a mental attitude is to simply keep your word to practice every day. Even a few minutes of Long, Deep Breathing is a yoga Sadhana. Whatever your inclination—whether you're comfortable starting simply or prefer to start right off with a more complex regimen—start a yoga regimen and practice it daily. Through this first stage, you will undoubtedly confront your ego and question your motivation and/or your abilities. Be sensitive to the ways you may try to sabotage your practice, and give yourself a chance! The reality of daily practice may at times seem quite challenging. In the beginning of this book, we described meditation as "taking out the garbage," a metaphor for eliminating thoughts that continuously interfere with your success or limit your potential. Taking out the garbage is not a blissful experience! At times, you will have to count on your commitment to persevere through any resistance you experience. At other times, you will rejoice as the self-healing aspects of yoga practice begin to liberate your energy and change your negative thought patterns. Yoga works!

After a period of time, you will move into the second stage of *Aradhana* (pronounced *ah-rah-dah-nah*). In Aradhana, you reach a new level of subconscious cleansing through your meditations. At times you may experience boredom or you may believe that you have already finished what you have set out to do. You may feel that you have accomplished something great and feel satiated. The trick at this stage of practice is to keep going! The process of self-healing has no end: The Divine Self is greater than any of us can know; there is always more positive growth to experience. As you continue your practice, you will inevitably discover more ways in which your mind is limiting your infinite potential, and your experience of the divine power within you will expand and deepen.

If you keep up through this tricky time, you can pass into the stage of *Prabupati* (pronounced *prah-boo-bah-tee*). This is the stage of crystallization, the stage at which you achieve mastery of the neutral yoga mind. Your motivation to practice is purely to experience the union of your true self with your physical being. Your practice is generated from the knowledge that it is your inner light, your self-love that gives you radiance—not any outside circumstances, superficial appearances, or physical abilities. This is a stage of awakening in which your senses are aware and you feel pain and pleasure but are motivated by neither. You operate in the world and simultaneously are not of it. The polarities of your desires do not distract you from maintaining the practice to experience your life fully. This entire process can take months or years, depending on many factors; each individual brings a unique history, temperament, and capacity for practice. The journey itself is worth the effort.

Practically speaking, it takes about forty days of daily practice to begin to break an old habit and replace it with a new one. Within a relatively short time, these new habits can create a new, healthier you. As with any discipline, strive to practice every day to heal the body, focus the mind, and uplift your spirit. Once you create the habit of yoga practice, the daily and cumulative benefits of this action will support you each day of your life. Here are some helpful hints to help you keep up:

When to Practice

It is best to practice yoga and meditation in the morning, before you start your day. Consider rising before the sun (called the "ambrosial hours" in yoga), when your energy is supportive of your practice and it is quiet and peaceful. Doing so honors your primary commitment to yourself and enables you to meet your day with strength and spirit. If practicing in the morning is not possible, fit it in whenever you can. Try attaching your yoga practice to another activity you do each day. For example, practice right before or after your morning shower or the first thing after work and before dinner, or right before bed, etc.

What to Wear

Practice yoga in comfortable clothing that is loose around your thighs and is made from a natural fiber. (We have illustrated the postures in this book with leotards and tights to help you see the postures clearly.) According to the ancient practice of Kundalini Yoga, your energy remains balanced when you maintain a pocket of air around your upper thighs and groin. This air pocket will balance the energy in your lower chakras and add to your vitality.

Where to Practice

Create a cozy place to practice. Ideally this space should have natural light and be well ventilated with fresh air. Set aside enough space on the floor in which to lie down and to stretch both up and down and side to side. For best results and comfort, use a natural mat or blanket made of cotton or wool. Practicing in the same place every day will also make it easier to maintain a yoga discipline. This sacred personal space—a spare room, or part of a room—can be a sanctuary for your soul and a place to honor your spirit and commitment.

How to Practice

In each chapter of *A Woman's Book of Yoga* you will see new exercises, postures, and meditations designed for specific situations. Remember to tune in with the mantra *Ong Naamo Guroo Dayv Naamo,* take a few moments to breathe and relax, and then begin your yoga practice. After you are done and have relaxed, sit up and take a moment to radiate a prayer for peace. Prayers and affirmations done at the end of yoga practice have great power. We end Kundalini Yoga classes with a positive affirmation and projection.

Your First At-Home Class

In the East, age was measured more by the flexibility and vitality of the spine than by the actual number of years lived. If your spine is flexible and your energy flows freely to the organs and glands in your body, you are considered to be young.

For this reason, spinal care and exercise are among the first practices of yoga. They should be done daily and gradually. You cannot force your spine to become flexible. Flexibility is a long-term goal and is achieved with practice. The following exercise set provides you with a foundation for enjoying all yoga and meditations and for beginning the practice of Kundalini Yoga. It is an excellent warm-up for more vigorous yoga sets and postures and also stands alone as a set to energize your entire system. This exercise series works systematically, from the base of the spine to the top, to keep your spine flexible and healthy. All twenty-six vertebrae, your chakras, and energy bodies receive stimulation and a burst of energy, which makes this series a good one to do before meditation.

As a beginner, you can take more time to integrate the effects of each exercise by extending the rest periods between exercises to 3 minutes. If you feel pain when you practice these exercises, see a professional, such as a chiropractor or osteopathic or orthopedic physician, for advice regarding restrictions on your exercise routine. Remember to choose the seated posture you can maintain most comfortably. If your legs get tired, take a break. Use a cushion or blanket, or remain seated in a chair. To review how to sit, how to breathe, or the other basics you will need to begin, refer to Chapter 2.

One last note: The postures and exercises in Kundalini Yoga are usually presented in sets, called *kriya*s, arranged in precise sequences in order to create certain effects. Their sequences should not be altered. Some exercises can be practiced individually, and they will be clearly marked throughout the book.

Step One: Tune In with *Ong Naamo Guroo Dayv Naamo*

Sit in Easy Pose, with your legs crossed, or in a comfortable seated posture. Bring your palms together in front of your rib cage. Bend your thumbs and

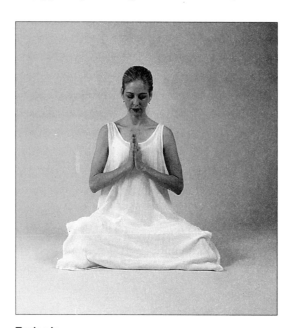

Tuning in

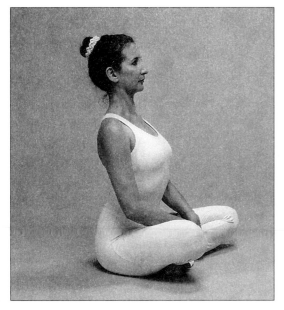

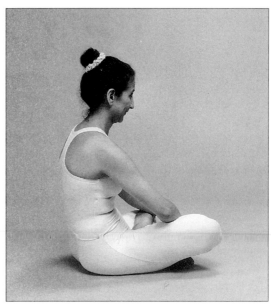

**Spinal flex showing inhalation and
forward motion in Easy Pose**

**Spinal flex showing exhalation and
backward motion in Easy Pose**

press the knuckles gently into your sternum. This is called Prayer Pose. Close your eyes and bring your awareness to your environment as you begin to create a sacred place for doing yoga. Then repeat the mantra for tuning in three times. Inhale and suspend your breath briefly. Exhale and relax.

Step Two: Pranayam

Remain sitting in a comfortable position. Relax your hands in your lap and practice Long, Deep Breathing for 3 minutes. Pay attention to all of your sensations as you breathe. Breathe fully and completely. To end, inhale and suspend your breath briefly. Exhale and relax.

Step Three: Basic Spinal Energy Kriya

1. *Spinal Flex in Easy Pose—Hold Ankles.* Sit in Easy Pose (cross-legged) and grasp your ankles with both hands. Inhale as you flex your spine forward and lift your chest up, arching your back forward. Exhale as you flex your spine backward and tilt your pelvis back. Keep

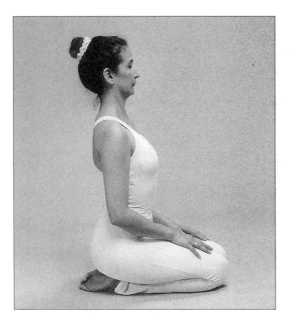

Spinal flex showing inhalation and forward motion in Rock Pose

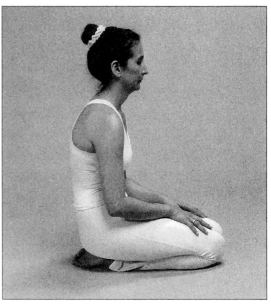

Spinal flex showing exhalation and backward motion in Rock Pose

your head and chin level, while keeping your neck relatively still. Concentrate on the movement of your spine and the rhythm of your breath and mentally chant *Sat* as you inhale and *Naam* as you exhale. Continue this movement 26–108 times. To end, inhale deeply and suspend (hold) your breath for 10–30 seconds. Concentrate your energy at your brow point just between your eyes. Then rest for 1 minute as you relax your breath, sit, and become still.

2. ***Spinal Flex in Rock Pose—Palms Down.*** Sit in Rock Pose. Place your hands flat, palms facing down, on your thighs. Flex your spine with the same breath and mantra rhythm as in the previous exercise. Continue 26–108 times. To end, inhale as you straighten your spine, suspend your breath, and focus at your brow point. Hold for 10–30 seconds. Relax for 2 minutes.

The Power of the Spinal Flex

The basic spinal flex is a magnificent exercise. In addition to helping you develop flexibility and relieve stiffness in your back, this exercise also massages your pelvic organs, which the yoginis consider a daily requirement for women. As you practice the spinal flex, concentrate on your lower back and pelvic area. Feel the nonforce massage you are giving your lower back, and then expand your awareness to include your whole spine.

The spinal flex also stimulates the flow of spinal fluid, which refreshes the brain and stimulates your nervous system to increase your energy and awareness. In fact, a study done by Neil Goodman, Ph.D., at the University of California at Davis (December 1973), showed that the spinal flex exercise created large changes in EEG activity during and after exercise. The exercise has a "multistage reaction pattern" that greatly alters the proportions and strengths of alpha, theta, and delta waves. By combining the repetition of the mantra with rhythmic, coordinated breathing, you will create a powerful effect in a very short time.

3. ***Spinal Twist in Easy Pose.*** Grasp your shoulders with your fingers in front, thumbs in back. Your right hand grasps your right shoulder, left hand, your left shoulder. Inhale as you twist to the left. Exhale and twist to the right. Twist from your navel point, keeping your head steady and twisting with your upper body. Stay relaxed during the motion. Continue 26–108 times. To end, inhale as you face forward. Hold 15–30 seconds. Relax for 1 minute.

4. ***Bear Grip Mudra—"Seesaw" Exercise.*** Sit in Easy Pose. Curl the fingers of each hand and hook them to each other, forming a lock in front of your chest, at the level of your heart, left palm out at the level of the heart center, right palm facing in toward the left palm. Lock your thumbs down on the little finger of the opposite hand. Move your elbows in a seesaw motion. Add deep, powerful breaths. It looks like a propeller. Continue 26 times. To end, inhale and exhale all your breath out. As you hold your breath out, tighten the Bear Grip by pulling your hands apart without breaking the grip, keeping your

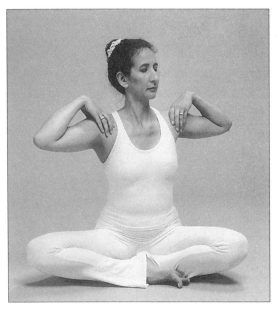

Spinal Twist

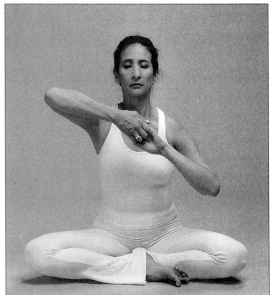

Seesaw exercise in Bear Grip Mudra

forearms parallel to the ground. Apply the Root Lock (*Mula Bhandha*) as described in Chapter 2. Relax for 30 seconds.

5. ***Spinal Flex, Easy Pose—Elbows Straight.*** In Easy Pose, grasp your knees firmly with your hands, keeping your elbows straight. Flex your spine using the breath and mantra, as in Exercise 1. With elbows straight, the flexing motion will automatically center on the upper spine and chest. Continue 26–108 times. Then inhale, hold, and concentrate at the brow for 10–30 seconds. Exhale and relax for 1 minute.

6. ***Light Shoulder Shrugs.*** Sit in Easy Pose. Lift both shoulders straight up in a shoulder shrug as you inhale. Your shoulders should feel lively and light, not tense and cramped. On the exhale let the shoulders drop back to their original posture. Continue at a pace of about 70–90 shrugs per minute. Your breath will be quick and shallow, as with Breath of Fire, creating a sniffing sound. Begin more slowly if you need to or take breaks as you build up your time. Continue for 2 minutes. Then inhale, lift the shoulders, and hold for 15 seconds. Exhale and relax.

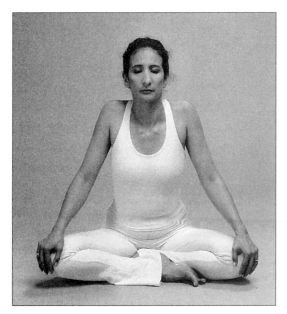

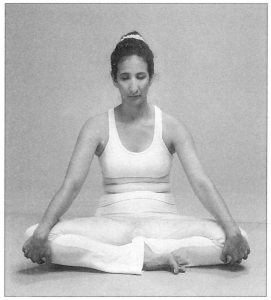

Spinal Flex with elbows straight, inhalation, and forward motion

Spinal Flex with elbows straight, exhalation, and backward motion

7. ***Neck Rolls.*** Remain in Easy Pose. Keep your spine straight. Roll your neck slowly to the right and back to center 5–10 times. Then roll it to the left 5–10 times. When you roll it, be careful to find a circular swing that matches the mobility of your neck. (The neck is not designed to roll evenly.) Then inhale deeply and pull the head and neck straight. Relax.

8. ***Bear Grip Mudra—Root Lock Exercise.*** Remain in Easy Pose. Raise your hands in front of your throat. Form the Bear Grip mudra, as in Exercise 4. Hold your elbows extended and parallel to the ground. Inhale deeply, exhale, inhale, and hold. Apply the Root Lock (*Mula Bhandha*), then exhale, inhale, and exhale completely. Hold it out and apply *Mula Bhandha*. Repeat this cycle three times. Then move the Bear Grip about 4 inches over the crown of the head. Repeat the breath and lock cycle three times. Then start back at the throat and repeat the entire cycle one more time.

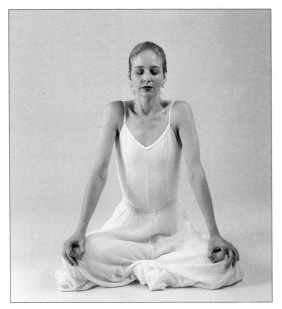

Light shoulder shrugs

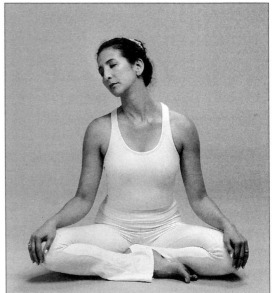

Neck rolls

9. ***Sat Kriya***—Sitting on your heels in Rock Pose, stretch your arms straight up and over your head, elbows hugging your ears. Interlace your fingers with your index fingers, stretching up. Your thumbs are crossed to hold your hands locked together. Keep your elbows as straight as you can. As you chant the word *Sat* aloud, pull the navel point (belly) in and up. As you chant the word *Naam* aloud, release the navel point and relax the belly. Continue chanting with a powerful projection. Each time you chant *Sat* and pull in your navel point area, you will feel your pelvic floor lift a bit. Create a steady rhythm of chanting, about eight *Sat Naam* repetitions per every 10 seconds. If you bring your attention to the sound and vibration of the mantra, your breath will adjust itself. Do not flex your spine. Concentrate on the mantra and the steady pulsing movement of your navel point area.

Continue chanting for 3–11 minutes. To end the exercise, inhale deeply and hold the breath in, without straining. Consciously apply the Root Lock, pulling in at the navel point and up on the sex organs and anal sphincter muscle, thus lifting the pelvic floor. Focus your

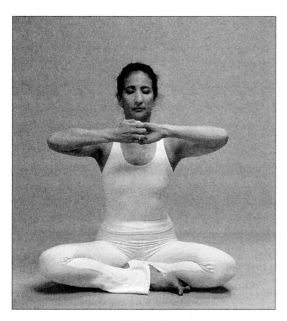

**Bear Grip Mudra—Root Lock exercise
with arms parallel to floor**

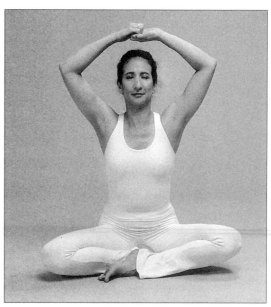

**Bear Grip Mudra—Rock Lock exercise
with arms above head**

eyes at your brow point. Hold for 5–10 seconds and exhale. Repeat this sequence two more times and then relax. After you complete Sat Kriya, it is best to relax for twice the amount of time that you practiced the exercise. This helps the energy stimulated by the exercise to become integrated into your body and mind.

You can practice this exercise alone or together with other postures or yoga kriyas. Begin your practice for 1–3 minutes and slowly build your time as your endurance and strength increase. With common sense and a steady practice, you can gradually build Sat Kriya up to 31 minutes.

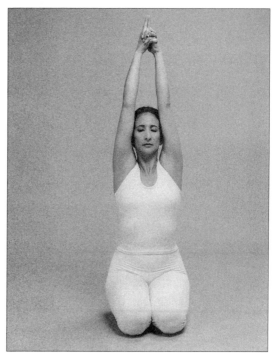

Sat Kriya

SAT KRIYA—VITALIZING AND CALMING

It is said that if you only have a few minutes to practice Kundalini Yoga, do Sat Kriya. Once learned, Sat Kriya is unmatched for increasing focus, concentration, and your core energy of awareness—the kundalini. As you rhythmically pulse your navel area, you strengthen your pelvic-floor muscles and create better health for sexuality and bladder control as well as stimulate your digestion. You also circulate the spinal fluid, which strengthens your nervous system and prolongs the life of neurons, effectively improving your mood and mood disorders and strengthening your individual projection.

Energetically, Sat Kriya synchronizes your mind, body, and soul, and creates new patterns of circulation throughout your entire system. This synchronization and stimulation signal your body and mind to wake up and experience your soul. Through this process you can gain tremendous stamina and strength, and can conquer chronic fears. And because this kriya awakens the energy of the first three chakras, you will have greater access to vitality, projection, and presence. As a woman, these qualities enable you to relax and stay centered.

Step Four: Meditation on the Chakras

The practice of yoga and meditation affects both your physical body and your Subtle Anatomy. This meditation will help you to locate each chakra in your body, to experience the vibration of each center, and to raise your energy.

Sit in Easy Pose or in any comfortable position with your spine straight. Inhale deeply. As you exhale, chant a long *Sat Naam*. The *a* in *Sat* is drawn out for almost the entire breath, with *Naam* chanted in a very short vibration at the very end of your exhalation: *Saaaaaaaaaaaaaaaaaaaaaaaaaaaaat Naam*.

As you exhale and chant, apply the Root Lock, or *Mula Bhandha,* and concentrate on the first chakra located at the rectum, the base of the spine—the center of security and grounding.

Release the Root Lock. Inhale deeply again, and concentrate on the second chakra, the reproductive and sex organs, including the vagina and ovaries—the center of creativity and flow. Applying the Root Lock, exhale and chant *Saaaaaaaaaaaaaaaaaaat Naam.*

Continue the sequence, inhaling and chanting while applying the Root Lock with each chakra:

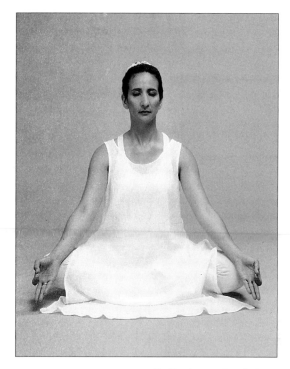

Meditation on the chakras

- Third Chakra: the Navel Point, solar plexus, digestion—center of power and will

- Fourth Chakra: the Heart Center, rib cage, thymus gland—center of compassion

- Fifth Chakra: the Throat Center, thyroid—center of communication and manifestation

- Sixth Chakra: the Third Eye or brow point—center of insight and intuition

- Seventh Chakra: the Crown Chakra, at the crown of your head—center of divine connection and cosmic vibration and sound

- Eighth Chakra: the Aura, the field of your impact and impression surrounding you in all directions—the center of projection and presence

You can repeat the sequence from the first to the eighth chakra many times. When you have completed a sequence, inhale and suspend your breath briefly. Exhale and relax.

Step Five: Relaxation in Corpse Pose

After you meditate, take a moment to enjoy the effects of your concentrated efforts. Lie on your back and relax. Support your neck with a rolled towel, if needed, and stretch your back by bringing your knees to your chest, if your back is stiff. Relax on your back, arms by your sides, palms facing upward.

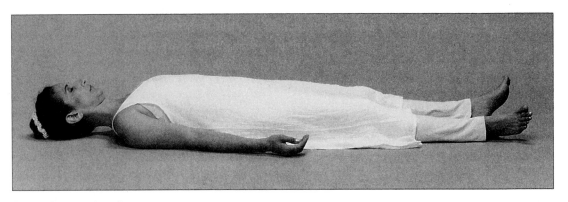

Corpse Pose—relaxation

Sense the echoes of your chanting in your physical body, in your mind, in your total being. Surrender: Let yourself go into that echo and be complete. Relax in this position for 3–11 minutes.

How to Relax

If you have difficulty relaxing, try the following techniques:

Focusing the Mind

Visualize the inside of your forehead as a movie screen. As you inhale, mentally see the mantra *Sat* written on the screen. As you exhale, visualize the mantra *Naam* written on the screen. Continue this visualization until your mind relaxes.

Progressive Relaxation

Bring your awareness to each muscle, organ, and gland—all the parts of your body. Start at your feet and move upward. As you bring your awareness to each muscle, you can tense it, and then let it go, mentally instructing it to relax. After you move through the major muscles, bring your awareness inward to your organs, glands, nerves, and bones. Gently invite each part of you to relax. Take your time and enjoy the benefits of directing kindness toward yourself.

"Lighten your load." Visualize yourself floating, weightless, above your body. Allow yourself to become like a bird, flying through the air, limitless and totally creative. Feel the sensations of flight, see the colors of the sky, and enjoy yourself flying fast or slow, high or low. Travel to a healing sanctuary. Your "healing sanctuary" can be a place you know or one you create. Feel free to wander and explore your healing sanctuary, taking in the experience with all your senses. When you return to the present moment, embody the healing experience and let it penetrate into every cell.

Science, Yoga Practice, and Well-Being

DR.'S NOTES

If you have been practicing yoga for a while, you probably already have experienced its benefits. But if you are a beginner, you are in for a treat! Healthy women who participate in yoga classes report greater life satisfaction and better ability to cope with stress. That is likely because they experience less excitability, aggressiveness, and emotionality and fewer somatic complaints.

When a group of forty-eight volunteers were tested using a standardized Subjective Well-Being Inventory (SUBI) after 4 months of practicing yoga, they had an overwhelming sense of improved well-being. These reports are not just a change in perspective. After just 4 weeks of yoga training, these women were able to exercise more comfortably with a lower heart rate and slower breathing. These findings were correlated with reduced oxygen consumption— that is, yoga helped the women in the study get into better shape. Women will be interested to know that even though both men and women benefit from yoga, the benefits are most pronounced in women.

Even if you are already in good condition, you can still look to yoga for additional benefits. A group of forty physical education teachers with an average of 8.9 years of physical training participated in 3 months of yogic training. They achieved a significant improvement in their general health as measured by weight loss, lowered blood pressure, and improved lung function. They also were found to have a more balanced autonomic nervous system with a slower heart rate and respiration, and increased steadiness.

Even conditioned athletes can lower their heart rate and rate of breathing, and their bodies can learn to use oxygen more efficiently through the practice of yoga. A group of exercisers were asked to use a treadmill to raise their heart rate and blood pressure. Immediately afterward, some of the volunteers were asked to simply rest, while the remainder performed yogic relaxation postures. The volunteers who used yoga had their blood pressure and heart rate return to normal much sooner than those who simply rested. These demonstrated changes offer excellent objective proof that yoga helps to synchronize the body and balance the autonomic nervous system. And these benefits are noticeable

 within weeks after beginning, even if you are already in good condition.

Twenty-Minute Easy Yoga Session

1. Tune in.

2. Practice Long, Deep Breathing for 1–3 minutes, then relax for 1–3 minutes.

3. Practice the spinal flex for 1–3 minutes.

4. Meditation on the chakras.

5. Relax.

6. Projection for peace, affirmation for healing.

One-Hour Yoga Session

1. Tune in.

2. Practice the basic spinal series, including Sat Kriya.

3. Relax.

4. Meditation on the chakras.

5. Projection for peace, affirmation for healing.

Practice either yoga session as listed above at different times of the day. Notice if there is any difference in practicing yoga at these times:

- Ambrosial hours of 4:00–6:00 A.M.
- Midday
- Evening between 4:00 and 6:00 P.M.
- Nighttime directly before you go to sleep

QUESTIONS FOR FURTHER GROWTH

- What sensations do you feel after your yoga session? Keep a journal and watch your progress as the exercises become more familiar to you.

- Does doing yoga at different times during your day have different effects?

- When is the best time to practice according to your current schedule and habits?

- Is there one time that you can commit to practice even a few minutes every day?

4

Your Moon Centers: Yogic Cycles and Transitions

Woman is the moon. It wanes and waxes. Everything grows because of the moon. Everything ripens because of sun. And everything is conceived because of the combination of the harmony and those two polarities of male and female, sun and moon.

—YOGI BHAJAN

Change is a constant part of life, both within us and in the larger pattern of nature. The seasons change in a regular rhythm, and the earth, moon, and planets constantly shift positions in the heavens. With each breath, your body systems also shift and adjust; with every thought you think and every movement you make, you create an effect, a change that moves you through time. Every seven years, every cell in your body is replaced with a new cell, creating in effect a totally new person. In every inch of the cosmos and within every living being, changes are constantly taking place. This process of constant change is part of the evolution of life and will continue forever.

The changes women commonly notice are the physical cycles their body goes through, such as the menstrual cycle. On a larger scale, the yogis describe the cycle of life and transition with the mantra *Saa Taa Naa Maa*, which means "birth, life, death, and rebirth." Every action you take and every thought you think has a birth, life (or existence), death (or transition), and leaves you newly affected or reborn. Living life consciously means constantly engaging in the process of change.

On many subtle levels, a woman's body manifests the creative, cosmic aspect of change. She does this in part through a specific cycle that develops when she is in the womb, just after conception. This cycle, called the Moon Center sequence, is the subtlest and most significant cycle a woman can sense and experience (see more details in the next section of this chapter). After the Moon Center cycle is fixed, and while her physical body is still developing in the womb, her menstrual cycle is determined. By the time a woman is born, she contains all the eggs in her ovaries that she will have for her entire life. Therefore, in a sense, despite any changes in her life due to health and self-care, her menopause is determined as well. When a woman is born, then, she is the physical manifestation of the universal *Adi Shakti,* the primal feminine energy; she reflects and embodies all the cycles of life.

When a woman resists change, especially the changes in her own body, it is like resisting her own nature. One of the basic teachings of yoga is for a woman to be a woman, for a woman to love herself as a woman, for a woman to accept herself as a woman. In other words, when a woman understands her own basic nature of cycle and transition, she finds power in that foundation. If we consider the metaphor of the feminine kundalini—the "coil," or the potential energy that is ready to transform, transition, and become creative at any moment—we can see that the power of potential and transition is the power of a woman to uplift herself and the world.

The ancient writings, as taught by Yogi Bhajan and discussed in this book, address each specific cycle of the feminine transitions. These teachings help you understand yourself; through this self-knowledge you can develop self-love, from which comes self-respect. The result of self-respect is the ability to respect all life and to direct the energy of your life toward your highest values and destiny.

Understanding Your Emotional Intelligence and Psyche

In the philosophy of Kundalini Yoga, women are often referred to as "lunar beings." As women go through their menstrual cycle, the natural world around them also cycles. Women have always been closely in touch with nature and with each other. It has been noted that women who live together tend to cycle together. Similarly, thousands of years ago, women who noticed the connection between their own cycles and the cycles of the moon created the ancient lunar calendar.

The phases of the moon have often been related to the phases of the menstrual cycle. Using this primal model, you can see that your body has a wisdom that evolves and changes throughout the month. Your physical cycles keep you aware of your fertility, your femininity, your strength, and your renewal. Each month is like a full phase of the moon, passing through cycles like the seasons of the year. Ovulation metaphorically correlates to a full moon, pregnant with possibilities and summer. After ovulation, you wane like the moon, moving through autumn into the dark of winter or your new moon, which is expressed as menstruation. Spring follows with the development of your maturing eggs as you wax toward ovulation and your full moon again.

Kundalini Yoga compares men to the sun, which is constant, and women to the moon, which fluctuates. As a woman who possesses the many qualities of the moon, you have the ability to reflect and absorb, wax and wane, create and nurture, release and renew, and be both subtle and strong. It is said that it takes a woman 14 days to wax and 14 days to wane, but a man does it with fourteen breaths waxing and fourteen breaths waning. This means that the man goes through the process in 2 minutes, the woman in 28 days. The outer, more noticeable difference is that the woman spends enough time in each Moon Center to experience the transition both within her mind and moods and in her actions. The man moves more quickly, sensing less transition and manifesting a more sunlike nature.

The special teaching for women that follows is more than six thousand years old and can help you understand and embrace your physical and emotional fluctuations.

The Eleven Moon Centers

The essence of a woman is moon in quality. —Yogi Bhajan

Ancient wisdom teaches that a woman has eleven Moon Centers. These centers are located in different parts of the body and relate directly to specific qualities that a woman uses to process her environment and emotions.

THE ELEVEN MOON CENTERS AND THE QUALITIES THEY REPRESENT

Hairline: the arc line—steadiness, stability, divine clarity, reality

Cheeks: unpredictability, emotional stability

Lips: verbal, interactive, communicative

Ear lobes: intelligence, concern with values and ethics

Back of the neck: sensitivity, romance

Breasts: divine compassion, giving (can be to the point of foolishness)

Belly button/Back: insecure, exposed, vulnerable

Inner thighs: confirmative, verifying, affirming

Eyebrows: illusionary, imaginative, visionary

Clitoris: external, talkative in social situations

Vagina: depth, sharing in personal or cultural cycle

These eleven Moon Centers are said to move within the body, revolving around the chin—the moon spot. Men naturally grow hair on their chins, which calms the moon effect. In some meditations, you may be asked to close your eyes and focus them downward, toward your chin. This eye focus helps calm the emotions and creates harmony and balance. Each woman has a unique path through which the Moon Centers cycle. Your psyche resides in each Moon Center, or waxes and wanes through different qualities, for $2\frac{1}{2}$ days. You complete the entire cycle in 28 days, roughly the same length of time as your menstrual cycle.

Your unique Moon Center pattern does not depend on the actual phase of the moon or your menstrual cycle. This cycle and model can explain many

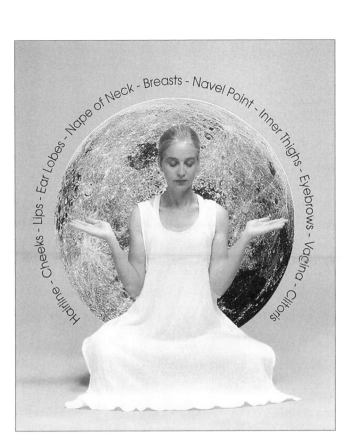

Hairline - Cheeks - Lips - Ear Lobes - Nape of Neck - Breasts - Navel Point - Inner Thighs - Eyebrows - Vagina - Clitoris

Moon Centers

patterns that have seemed so mysterious to us in the past. Women have been labeled as unpredictable, always changing their minds, always delivering the unexpected day to day. Women have been compared to witches and shape shifters, and are thought to have great powers of transformation. Secretly, and publicly, cultures have both revered and repressed the waxing and waning nature of women.

Every 2½ days, when you cycle to a different Moon Center, you see the world through the quality of that center. As your Moon Center changes, your mood will change. If you are aware of your Moon Center, you can feel the tug of that quality. During the 2½ days in that particular Moon Center, you will apply that certain quality to your projects and ideas, to your creativity. Your Moon Center cycle stays with you throughout your entire life, although it may be more evident to you at different times of life.

The Menstrual Cycle and Your Moon Centers

When a young woman begins to menstruate, the power of the cycle of menstruation and ovulation can be intense. Many women have reported feeling a desire for sex right before and during ovulation (some women feel this very strongly), feeling moody right before menstruation begins, and having the desire for solitude during the first days of flow. The sexual drive is naturally connected to the menstrual cycle. On certain days of the month your body is more receptive to conception and on others to projection. Although your Moon Centers cycle continuously through your menstrual cycle, during youth and prime times for conception, a woman may feel her menstrual cycle connection more strongly. The power of your desire manifests through the Moon Center you are in. Clearly the layers of cosmic, mental, and physical cycling are amazingly complex!

Mapping Your Moon Center Pattern

Understanding your Moon Center pattern gives you insight into your emotional flow. It benefits you to track this patterned cycling of your emotional status and psyche. Understanding your unique pattern can provide a compass for your primal creative and intuitive nature, as it reflects your capacity to be creative, process ideas and situations, and manifest your ideas and projects while always seeing the big picture.

Your Moon Centers and your sexuality are also connected. The yogis teach that you are more sexually sensitive in the area of your present Moon Center. There is an ancient painting that illustrates the Moon Centers, indicated by the "traveling" of the God Kama—the god of pleasure—through the body. There were instructions in Sanskrit on how to understand these centers of pleasure. If you are in an active sexual relationship, you can also locate your Moon Center by exploring your centers during foreplay and finding where you are most sensitive. It can be a lot of fun having your partner "chase down" your Moon Center and become sensitive to your mood and your body (see Chapter 6 for more information on "Moon Centers and Sexuality").

It takes some time and sensitivity to track your Moon Centers and determine your particular sequence. Watch how you are feeling each day for a few months, making special note of the general descriptions of the Moon Centers and their qualities. After a few months your pattern will become clear. If the pattern is not clear, practice the meditations recommended to enhance your sensitivity and help balance all of the Moon Centers.

Here is an example of what a pattern for a woman's Moon Centers might look like:

Hairline: reality
Ear lobes: values
Inner Thighs: confirmative
Belly button/Back: insecure, vulnerable
Back of the neck: romantic
Lips: verbal
Cheeks: unpredictable
Breasts: compassionate
Eyebrows: illusionary
Vagina: sharing in personal or cultural cycles
Clitoris: external, talkative in social situations

For instance, if this woman is in the Moon Center of her neck one morning, she feels very open and romantic and buys flowers on the way to work. While she's walking down the street, she notices that the man and woman normally waiting for the bus are talking and laughing, maybe even amorously, and she contemplates this. She notices the beauty of the gardens and flowers. She can smell the scents of her neighborhood particularly well today and is ready for an adventure. She smiles. Everything runs smoothly, and she is in no rush to go anywhere.

The next morning she awakens in the Moon Center of the lips. She can't wait to tell her friend about the news report last night and calls before breakfast. She talks until she is a bit late. After running for the bus, she joins the conversation at the bus stop and enjoys connecting with others. She says hello to the bus driver and asks the time; it is easier than looking at her watch.

You may notice that you, too, experience this type of mood shift. One day you feel like talking all the time; the next day you want to read and relax in the tub. It helps for you to know your pattern. If you do, you can understand your own psyche better and act accordingly. For instance, if you're having the tendency to be talkative, make sure you also listen, or seek out social times with friends. There is no need to judge which Moon Center you prefer, or where you would rather be. As a woman, you include them all.

If a woman experiences a trauma, the Moon Center pattern can change. For example, if the woman in the above example sees or is victim to a violent act when she is in the belly and feeling insecure, her Moon Center can change. She can move immediately from her belly to her hairline and automatically become sensitive in her own reality, or it can change to her breasts, as she becomes compassionate.

There are also situations in which women do not seem able to sense certain Moon Centers. As a result of stress or habits formed while young, a woman can totally repress one or more aspects of herself. For example, a woman can feel that she is never romantic or perhaps that she is never out of control or does not like to socialize. These can be coping mechanisms that she uses to protect herself. As a woman builds internal strength and self-respect, she needs fewer limiting coping mechanisms. Her internal strength allows for the manifestation of all her aspects.

In the business of new life, a woman can develop the habit of ignoring her own qualities, or preferring certain qualities to others. These choices are usually based on culturally defined judgments. A woman is deep and has both a direct and indirect nature, both light and shadow, like the moon. Her power comes from both the light and the shadow, from both her hidden and apparent faculties, if she learns how to process these two areas and flow with herself. With self-love and self-respect, both shadow and light create the alchemy of real creativity. The power of that energy directed toward Good and Love is unmatched.

Knowing the source of your power gives you the ability to deeply understand your own nature and make the best of your life. Know yourself as a woman. Respect yourself as a woman. Love yourself as a woman. Your reality will then become your grace and power.

Kirtan Kriya—Meditation to Balance Your Eleven Moon Centers

Kirtan Kriya is the meditation both for balancing your Moon Centers and for helping you go through transitions with strength and stability. The first version is specifically for women; both men and women can practice the second version. Kirtan Kriya is also a healing meditation for women trying to let go of past relationships with men, and is helpful in eliminating both the physical and mental associations with these men. Kirtan Kriya can give a woman a brilliant internal radiance that illuminates her aura and presence. Chose one version of Kirtan Kriya to practice according to your needs.

Kirtan Kriya—Balancing the Moon Centers and Glandular System

Lie on your stomach and place your chin on the floor. Keep your head straight, without looking left or right. Place your arms alongside your body, with the palms of the hands facing upward.

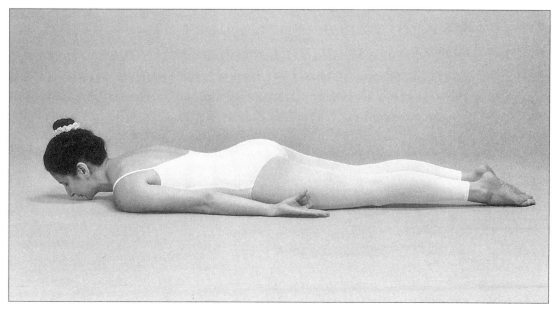

Kirtan Kriya—meditation to balance the Moon Centers

The mantra for this meditation, *Saa Taa Naa Maa*, is called the *Panj Shabad*. These basic syllables are the primal sounds of the mantra *Sat Naam*, the seed mantra of Truth. Each sound creates a unique vibration in your body and mind. These vibrations have the effect of stimulating a particular state of mind, as indicated by their meanings, which follow:

Saa—infinity, cosmos, beginning, and birth
Taa—life, existence
Naa—death, totality, and transition
Maa—rebirth, resurrection

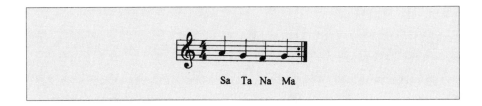

Sa Ta Na Ma

Chant the mantra silently, while focusing your eyes at your brow point. Meditate on the sound current (the mentally chanted mantra) coming in through the crown (top) of your head and flowing out through the center of the forehead (third eye point), creating an L shape.

As you mentally repeat the vibration of *Saa*, press your index finger to the tip of your thumb; on *Taa*, press your middle finger to your thumb; on *Naa*, press your ring finger to your thumb; and on *Maa*, press your little finger to your thumb. When you press each finger to your thumb, use enough pressure to really feel the connection. This helps keep you awake and in rhythm. Begin repeating the mantra and hand movements again, starting with *Saa*. Allow your breath to relax and regulate itself. Continue in this manner from 3 to 31 minutes.

Benefits Kirtan Kriya is significant for all women, as it is considered the highest meditation for a woman and should be done before any other meditation on earth. The mantra *Saa Taa Naa Maa* reflects the wheel of life. As you move your fingers in this particular way, you balance your brain and the different qualities of your personality. Each time you touch your finger to your thumb, for instance, you seal, balance, and integrate the qualities of infinity, beginning, and birth into your whole being. This meditation can also help you break any habit and assist you in going through any transition or change and its accompanying emotional turmoil. It is one of the most creative and beneficial meditations you can do.

Kirtan Kriya chanted in the belly position with your chin on the floor balances your Moon Centers. Start slowly and rest your head to one side if your neck becomes stiff.

Kirtan Kriya—Meditation for Strength and Stability Through Change

Sit in Easy Pose or in a chair with your feet flat on the floor. Repeat the mantra *Saa Taa Naa Maa* while using your fingers, as in the previous Moon Center meditation. Also use the visual process of repeating the mantra from the crown of your head through your brow point in an L shape.

Begin repeating the mantra aloud in a rhythmic way. Continue repeating the mantra aloud for 5 minutes. Then begin repeating the mantra in a whisper for 5 minutes. Next repeat the mantra silently for 10 minutes. Keep using your fingers while you repeat the mantra silently. After 10 minutes of silent repetition, whisper for 5 minutes, and then repeat aloud for 5 minutes. After you complete this last repetition segment, inhale and exhale deeply as you stretch your arms up as far as possible, spreading your fingers wide, for 1 minute. Then relax.

If you're just beginning to practice this meditation, you can shorten the times to 2 to 3 minutes for each cycle of chanting aloud, in a whisper, and silently. Then build gradually to the full 31 minutes. With patience, dedication, and common sense, you can build this meditation to 2½ hours.

Benefits This meditation is a jewel. When you chant aloud, you relate to the realm of the earth and to humanity. When you whisper, you relate to the realm of lovers, longing to belong and relate. When you chant silently, you relate to the realm of the divine and of infinity, beyond time and space. By chanting in all three voices, you can achieve a harmonious balance among body, mind, and soul.

Physically, yogis believe Kirtan Kriya stimulates your pituitary and pineal glands, which become active and balanced. Mentally, the meditation can eliminate negative thought patterns. Kirtan Kriya can help a woman release deeply held impressions of past negative sexual encounters. In this way, this mediation can help cleanse her aura and heal her from the trauma. On the subtle, spiritual level, you can stimulate a bright radiance and a powerful presence.

Meditation for Balancing Your Eleven Moon Centers

1. Tune in.

2. Long, Deep Breathing for 3 minutes; Segmented Breathing for 3 minutes; Breath of Fire for 1–3 minutes.

3. Spinal flex and Spinal twist.

4. Kirtan Kriya. Try each format: (1) On your stomach for balancing the Moon Centers; (2) sitting and using all three voices (aloud, whisper, and silent); and (3) chanting aloud for a few minutes.

5. Relax on your back for 11 minutes. If you are feeling insecure, relax for a few minutes on your belly as well; turn over onto your back when you want to and finish your relaxation.

QUESTIONS FOR FURTHER GROWTH

- Review the qualities of each of the eleven Moon Centers. Which Moon Center do you think you are in now?

- Map your moods and Moon Centers for a month. Take a few minutes each morning and at the end of each day to meditate, relax, and evaluate your location and sequence. Keep the map for several months and see if you can find a pattern.

- How do you act if your energy doesn't match what you have to do during the day? Do you create emotional resistance and negativity? Can you access the energy of that mood, relax, and transform it and apply it to the task at hand, or reschedule and remain in the flow of your day?

- How can understanding your Moon Centers help you with your relationships, your professional life, and your creativity?

5

Menstruation: Caring for Your Body, Mind, and Moods

Just remember, it is a simple habit to live in balance. Whenever you make a move, find out where the balance is and act accordingly.

—YOGI BHAJAN

The health of your menstrual cycle depends on your ability to relax. Stress accumulates daily and can cause exhaustion, depression, and, in extreme cases, disease. According to the teachings of Kundalini Yoga, the first place that stress manifests in a woman's body is in her ovaries. When a woman experiences continuous high levels of stress and does not have the techniques to recover and relax, her menstrual cycle may become imbalanced. Stress can cause too little or too much bleeding, late periods, or, in some cases, missed periods. When your period is out of balance, you are being signaled to evaluate your stress level, find ways to manage your stress, and bring balance into your life.

The yogic lifestyle, which includes a balanced diet, adequate exercise, and regular intervals of relaxation and meditation, is the best antidote to the stresses of modern life. Meditation in particular is a tremendously important tool for stress management. You cannot control the world around you, but regular meditation can help you control your own reactions to it. Your *reactions* to the negative circumstances of your life are the primary causes of stress.

Your menstrual cycle has physiological, psychological, and spiritual significance. Physiologically, it is the foundation for the transitions into womanhood, motherhood, and menopause, the beginning of the wisdom years. How you feel about your body can affect the health of your cycle. For too many young women, the desire to attain unreasonably thin figures can cause eating disorders or overexercising. Overeating, excessive sugar, caffeine from coffee or soft drinks, or imbalanced diets also affect overall health and the health of your cycle. If these long-standing negative habits are not addressed, they can cause irreversible and long-term damage to your body.

The physiological transitions that are marked by changes in the menstrual cycle, such as puberty, pregnancy, and menopause, correspond directly with times of spiritual transition. Ancient cultures often ritually celebrated these major spiritual events. In one Middle Eastern tradition, the entire community of women would gather and celebrate when a young woman began menstruating. At this celebration, the young girl would sit in the center of a circle and the wise women would dance around her. After the dance, the young girl could ask any question of any of the women. They would share wisdom and stories, and support the girl's transition into womanhood.

Yoga students in their teens report having little or no information on menstruation, and certainly no celebration or discussions of the psychological and spiritual importance of this event. Their periods are embarrassing and secret events that hold only one meaning—that they need to use birth control to avoid pregnancy. Without the deeper spiritual meaning, the menstrual cycle loses its significance. The original innocence, self-love, and curiosity of a young girl can be stifled by secrecy and result in a gender identity crisis, especially if the defining factor of becoming a woman becomes a negative event! It is not surprising that a negative view of the body leads young women to feelings of low self-esteem, isolation, and depression.

When you practice yoga and pay attention to your body, you are giving yourself permission to appreciate yourself and develop a more meaningful and positive relationship with your body. Practicing relaxation and meditation gives you the opportunity to experience your true identity—*Sat Naam*—and helps to transform negative patterns of thinking and acting. Every woman has a right to claim her Divine Self. All a woman has to do is appreciate, accept, and love herself as a woman, and the power will be hers!

Balancing Your Overall Cycle with a Yogini Lifestyle

The suggestions that follow will help keep you healthy the weeks before, during, and after menstruation.

Observe the times you experience an extra sensitivity, either 1 week or so before or after your period so you can adjust your lifestyle accordingly using the yoga in this chapter.

Learn to relax. Two 11-minute relaxation naps per day can train your body to recover from daily stress. Napping or deep relaxation will help keep your glandular system healthy.

Exercise daily. Include daily walks as part of your routine. Train yourself to practice the yoga exercises for women, and meditate to calm your mind.

Practice cold shower therapy, except during your menstrual period and pregnancy, for improved circulation and glandular health. Avoid quick hot showers; according to Kundalini Yoga, they are bad for the skin and for your cycle (see the section "Hydrotherapy" in Chapter 11).

Supplement your daily diet with raw oils. Taking raw oils is a common yogic prescription for women. Raw oils contain unsaturated fat and can also serve as a mild laxative when taken at night. One ounce of almond oil, if you are over the age of twenty-eight, can reduce hunger, keep your skin healthy, reduce body fat, and clear toxins from your system. One tablespoon of sesame oil twice daily can be added a few days before, during, and 4–5 days after menstruation to eliminate weakness and fatigue. You can take it with a little honey in milk.

Eat a balanced diet and take vitamin/mineral supplements. Healthy menstruation requires sufficient amounts of vitamins B, C, E, and folic acid, calcium, and magnesium as well as replacement amounts of iron due to loss of blood during menstruation. Although the total amount of blood lost is only a few ounces, supplemental iron can help prevent iron deficiency anemia. Check with your doctor before adding an iron supplement. Most women do not get all the vitamins and minerals they need from their diet and would benefit from a daily multivitamin. Also, those experiencing premenstrual syndrome (PMS) may benefit from calcium and magnesium supplements.

Avoid drastic diets that include fasting, unless you have prepared yourself ahead of time or are working with a medical provider's support. Drastic diets and fasting can disturb your glandular balance by depriving you of the necessary amounts of proteins and fats to manufacture hormones. Fasting can also deprive you of the essential vitamins and minerals that make your body work and protect you from certain diseases.

Take 2 tablespoons of turmeric every week. Turmeric helps you keep your vaginal and mucous membranes healthy. Turmeric is best taken cooked. Add a teaspoon to a bit of warm oil to form a sticky paste. You can also add ½ cup of turmeric to 1 cup of water. Heat the mixture until it forms a paste. Refrigerate the paste and take a take a small amount daily as a supplement. You can also add this spice to your foods.

Massage your breasts, lower back, and abdomen (ovaries) daily. Massaging these areas relieves tension and helps you relax. (This is especially effective before getting out of bed in the morning, but it can be done any time.) To stimulate your immune system and to calm your nervous system, massage your armpits for up to 20 minutes. Self-massage is an easy, self-healing modality and has many positive benefits.

Learn how to manage your feelings and process your emotions in appropriate ways. Work to avoid extended periods of extreme emotional states such as anger and tension, which can upset your menstrual cycle.

Establish a safe environment for you and your family. Women who are in an abusive relationship are in a struggle for survival. Physical, sexual, and/or emotional abuse may directly affect a woman's menstrual cycle as well as every other aspect of her life. Seek support or intervention if you need it. Do not permit yourself or your children to live in a negative or abusive environment.

Develop a positive self-image. Feelings of insecurity can lead to anxiety and depression, or to self-abuse through drugs, alcohol, or food. The practice of yoga and meditation will provide self-knowledge, self-acceptance, and a strong foundation for positive self-esteem, which will translate into healthier habits.

Ovulation

Hot baths. Take a hot bath during the few days of ovulation and sweat for 31 minutes. After the bath, cool off with a cold shower (be careful not to get dizzy). This therapy can help minimize problems and discomfort during your period.

While You're Menstruating

Here are some general suggestions to keep you healthy during menstruation.

Get help for menstrual irregularities. Pain, cramping, heavy bleeding, spotting, and missed periods suggest problems that require medical attention. Unchecked heavy bleeding can lead to anemia. Excessive fatigue and hypersensitivity to cold and heat, together with abnormal menstrual flow, may indicate thyroid disease. Menstrual irregularities may also indicate an unplanned or abnormal pregnancy. If you notice any of these symptoms, see your medical provider.

Improve menstrual cramps with calcium, magnesium, and exercise. In addition to having sufficient amounts of calcium and magnesium in your diet and regular exercise, regularly practice the four exercises that help prevent cramps (see the next section, "Yoga Postures for Menstrual Health").

Add ginger, garlic, or onion to your diet. In yogic tradition, these three roots are valued for their healing properties. When menstruation is very heavy, your nervous system can benefit from including ginger in your diet. When your flow is irregular, garlic is the root to add, as long as it doesn't cause gas. If you are anemic, onions can be helpful in addition to iron and B-complex vitamins.

Avoid excess salt to minimize water retention.

Avoid lifting heavy weight during your heaviest days of flow. Because your lower back is more sensitive during menstruation, heavy lifting can adversely affect the alignment of your hips and back, and cause back pain.

Eat six to ten almonds daily. Almonds provide energy, protein, magnesium, calcium, phosphorus, and potassium, as well as folic acid and vitamin E. If you eat them raw, first soak them and remove the skins to ease digestion. If you sauté them, you can eat the skins. (If you like, you can eat the sautéed almonds while they are warm.) Try eating almonds each morning of your menstrual flow for their nutritional benefit and to satisfy your cravings for fats and sweets.

Keep your diet light during menstruation. While your hormones are changing, a heavy diet will add stress to your body, so be sure to eat light.

Avoid medical procedures and undue stress during your menstrual cycle, when studies suggest that your resistance and immune system are at their weakest. Peak immunity is believed to be just before ovulation, and immunity in the first 2 weeks of the cycle is believed to be greater than in the last 2 weeks.

Take lukewarm showers. Avoid cold shower therapy.

Include daily activities that uplift your soul. During menstruation you may require more privacy and alone time. Take the opportunity to slow down and reflect. Use the occasion of menstruation for a monthly renewal of your mind and spirit.

Right after menstruation, resume your exercise schedule and include foods in your diet that are high in calcium, magnesium, and fiber.

DR.'S NOTES

The Science of Your Menstrual Cycle

Reproduction is one of the true miracles of the human body—a small bit of divinity within each woman that allows her to create life through loving union with her partner. As Charlotte the spider stated in E. B. White's *Charlotte's Web*, it is a magnum opus.

A woman's menstrual cycle begins when she herself is a fetus within her mother's uterus. At as early as 8 weeks of gestation, small germ cells destined to become eggs migrate through her developing body to areas that later will be transformed into ovaries. These cells begin to multiply rapidly, going from hundreds and thousands to more than 7 million by mid-pregnancy. Her developing brain releases large amounts of follicle-stimulating hormone (FSH) to levels that will not be reached again until she enters menopause. These primitive egg cells become surrounded by many layers of ovary cells that nurture and protect each egg and that will one day produce estrogen and progesterone, hormones necessary to prepare the uterine lining for the possibility of implanting a fertilized egg. By birth, the number of eggs dwindles to some 400,000. Given that there are roughly 360 menstrual cycles, there are more than enough eggs present for most women to conceive.

The brain's hormones enter a quiet phase at birth, dropping to baseline levels, and the immature eggs lie dormant for more than a decade. With the approach of puberty, higher centers of the brain awaken and hormone levels begin to rise, at first during sleep and later during both the day and night. Silent ovaries also awaken, and eggs that have been resting for more than a decade practice their ability to produce estrogen and progesterone in precise amounts and patterns. Hormone levels soar and plunge in anticipation of creating a first menstrual cycle. Hormones overshoot and undershoot until they get the levels right, in the meantime creating acne, mood swings, increased sexual interest, poor concentration, and confusion about body image. Pubic and underarm hair develops, breasts enlarge and firm up, and the uterine lining sheds irregularly in response to hormonal fluctuations. Once matured, a woman's exquisitely complex hormonal fluctuations synchronize into the menstrual cycle, coordinating the monthly selection and development of a mature egg with a perfectly prepared uterine lining, capable of receiving a fertilized egg, nurturing it, and allowing it to complete the cycle of life with the birth of a new child.

Stress-induced faulty ovulation is common in modern society. Often it is the result of inescapable exposure to multiple stresses: full-time work, doctors' appointments, poor relationships, financial survival, frequent travel—all combined with a lack of adequate support that leads to exhaustion and burnout. Reproductive hormones shut down, or their orderly release is disrupted, frequency of intercourse is reduced, and the potential for pregnancy is eroded. In addition, nerves from the brain that travel through the spinal cord directly to the reproductive organs can cause abnormal ovulation or reduced conception as a result of faulty movement of the fallopian tubes. Prolonged stress in menstruating women can also lead to an increased rate of bone loss.

In studies that I conducted with my colleagues Alice Domar and Herbert Benson at the Mind Body Program of Harvard Medical School, fifty-four in-

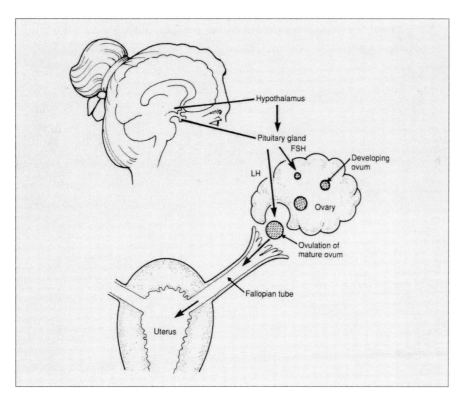

The Mind-Body Connection of Reproduction

fertile women who were enrolled in a behavioral treatment program were found to have increased levels of stress. For ten weekly meetings they were taught techniques for reducing stress and tension. They were also told to practice stress reduction at home for at least 20 minutes, twice a day. By the end of the program, they were significantly less anxious, depressed, and fatigued than before. In addition, 34 percent of these women became pregnant within 6 months of completing the program. Women who were infertile for a relatively short time (2.5 years on average) had a significantly higher rate of conception than those who were infertile for longer (an average of 3.5 years). This pattern is often seen with other infertility treatments as well. I am confident that similar studies conducted with yoga would yield similar results.

Yoga is a powerful tool, and regular practice can help you stay in the flow of your balanced menstrual cycle. The following yoga postures can help you keep your menstrual cycle healthy. Practice them throughout your life and whenever you sense that your cycle is out of balance. Take a few minutes to tune in, practice breathing exercises, and warm up your spine with the Spinal Flex and Spinal Twist before practicing any of the more rigorous postures.

Yoga Postures for Menstrual Health

Tiger Stretch

Sit on your right heel and extend your left leg straight behind you without bending your knee. Stretch up and let your head comfortably stretch back in alignment with the arch of your back. Even as you arch your back, keep stretching up so you do not compress your lower back too much. Bend your arms with your elbows as close to the sides of your body as possible. Place your hands at shoulder height facing the sky. If you are a beginner, hold the posture as long as you can. The goal is to hold this posture for 5 minutes with Long, Deep Breathing. Repeat the exercise stretching your right leg back.

Benefits Tiger Stretch opens circulation to your reproductive organs by releasing tension in the lower back. This can prevent menstrual cramps and painful menstruation. This exercise can also support the functions of your ovaries and kidneys, help you cleanse your liver, balance your hormones,

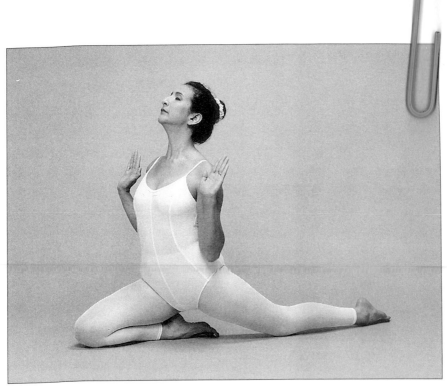

Tiger Stretch

and prepare you for the changes that occur in menopause. Don't wait for menopause to practice this exercise. Include it in your yoga routine so you can get the benefits from it now as well as later.

Half-Wheel Pose

Lie down on your back. Grab your ankles and draw your heels to the buttocks, with the heels about 18 inches apart. Tighten your buttock muscles, raise your entire torso up off the ground, and arch your spine, as if pressing your navel point to the sky. Hold this position for up to 3 minutes with Long, Deep Breathing. Slowly come down, stretch out your legs, and relax.

Benefits This exercise helps to strengthen your lower back, which can ache during your menstrual period. It also massages your reproductive organs and gives you strength. To release tension and massage your back any time you

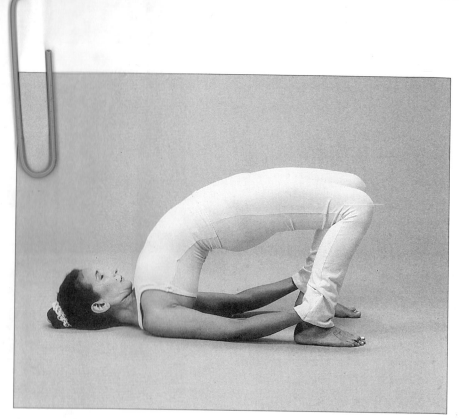

Half-Wheel Pose

need to, repeat this exercise twenty-six times, inhaling as you stretch up and exhaling as you relax down.

For Relief from Menstrual Cramps

The following exercises are a yoga prescription for relieving menstrual cramping. When practicing these exercises, use a deep, relaxing breath. Also take time to consciously and fully relax on your back for 3 minutes or more after each exercise. Practice each exercise alone or as a set.

Cobra Pose

Lie on your belly. Place your hands under your shoulders with your elbows by your side. Inhale as you lift your head and shoulders, pressing your hips into the floor and tightening your buttock muscles. Using your hands as sup-

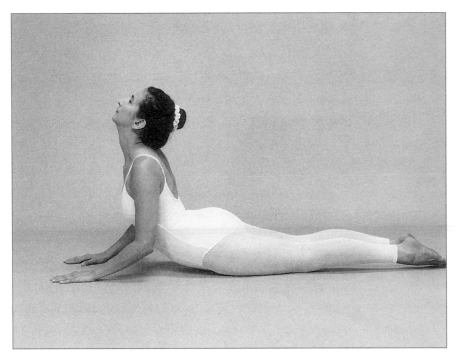

Cobra Pose

port, arch your back up, keeping your feet as close together as possible. Gently stretch your neck and focus on a point on the ceiling with Long, Deep Breathing or Breath of Fire for 1 minute.

Benefits Cobra Pose massages your ovaries and reproductive organs, maintains healthy circulation, and stretches your spine. This pose also massages your kidneys and can help relieve headaches (especially headaches due to improper diet). Practiced after the Half-Wheel Pose, Cobra Pose will stretch your entire spine and send healing energy circulating throughout your body.

Bow Pose

Lie on your stomach with your chin on the floor. Bend your knees and grasp your ankles. Tighten your buttocks and press your hip bones into the floor as you arch up, raising the thighs and head off the floor. Hold the position with Long, Deep Breathing for 2–3 minutes.

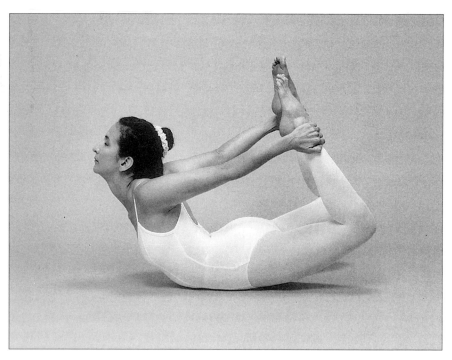

Bow Pose

Bow Pose Variation—Swan Salutation (*Hans Pranaam*)

Do this variation only if Bow Pose is easy for you and you can hold it for at least 1 minute. Once you are in Bow Pose, roll forward and back on your stomach up to 108 times, counting aloud. This is a rigorous variation that will make you sweat and massages your entire system.

Benefits Bow Pose is a full stretch for your spine. Feel the stretch across your belly and chest as you arch up. Bow Pose stimulates the flow of spinal fluid, refreshing your brain. Bow Pose is said to be powerful enough to help you adjust your mood right on the spot.

Beginner's Locust Pose

Lie on your stomach. Make your hands into fists and place them under your hips, just above the groin. Hold your heels together. Bring your attention to your lower back. Keeping your chin on the floor, and your shoulders relaxed,

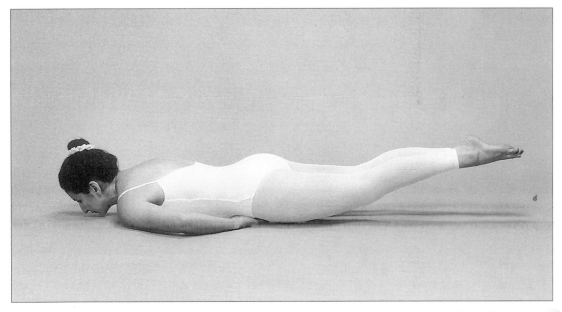

raise your legs off the floor. Hold this posture with Long, Deep Breathing for 1–2 minutes.

Benefits Locust Pose strengthens your lower back. This can be a rigorous pose when done correctly. Try to keep your upper body relaxed, using the strong muscles of your lower back to contract and lift the legs. As a beginner, your legs may only come up a few inches, and your feet may move apart from each other. Do your best to keep up!

Leg Lift

Lie on your back. Bring your heels together and raise your legs up at a forty-five-degree angle from the floor while keeping your legs straight. Hold this posture for up to 3 minutes with Long, Deep Breathing. Then relax your legs to the floor and become still in Corpse Pose with Long, Deep Breathing.

Benefits The Leg Lift exercises can be strenuous. They are frequently used to strengthen the back and abdominal muscles as well as to target particular organs and glands in the body (depending on the length of your legs). For

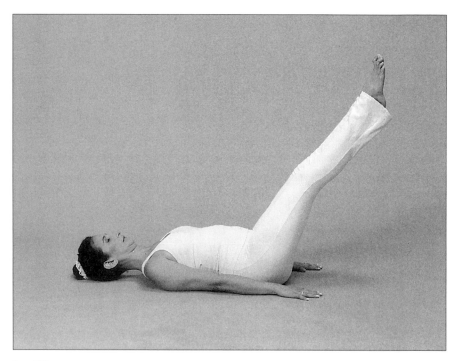

Leg Lift

extra support, you can place your hands under your lower back. If your back is tense after you finish and lower your legs to the floor, bring your knees to your chest and let your back relax before stretching out your legs. This particular exercise helps your liver, digestion, and elimination by working the muscles, meridians, nerves, and circulation associated with your digestive system.

Meditations

Breath Meditation to Regulate Menstrual Cycle

This is a gentle meditation technique to relieve mental fatigue and promote glandular balance. You can practice it any time you experience menstrual irregularities. Sit in Easy Pose with your legs crossed, or in a chair with your feet flat on the floor. Relax your arms and rest your wrists on your knees with your palms facing upward. Inhale through your nose in four segments. As you inhale, press your index finger to your thumb on the first inhaled segment, your middle finger to your thumb on the second inhaled segment, your ring finger to your thumb on the third inhaled segment, and your little finger to your thumb on the fourth inhaled segment. Mentally chant and meditate on the sounds of *Saa, Taa, Naa, Maa,* each sound matching one segment of breath as you inhale. Exhale in one long, continuous breath. Continue breathing in this rhythm for 3 minutes. Keep your eyes closed and your spine straight. To end the meditation, inhale deeply, suspend the breath, apply the Root Lock (see Chapter 2 for review), and hold briefly. Then exhale and relax.

Practice this meditation daily, increasing 1 minute per day until you are practicing the meditation for 7 minutes. Continue to practice 7 minutes daily for a week or so and then increase it again by 1 minute per day until you are meditating for 31 minutes, the maximum time for this meditation. You can then continue to practice it for 31 minutes daily.

Benefits The four-part breathing in this meditation brings your pituitary and pineal glands into a normal and healthy rhythm. This meditation can also help you erase and release negative thought patterns and achieve a clear, radiant, outer projection. When your inner and outer projections are positive and strong, your menstrual cycle can achieve balance.

Alternate Nostril Breathing

Sit in Easy Pose or in a chair with your feet flat on the floor. Hold your left hand in Gyan Mudra, resting on your knee. Use your right thumb to close your right nostril as you inhale through your left nostril. When you reach a full inhalation, use the index finger of your right hand to close your left nostril and remove your thumb to open your right nostril. Exhale through your right nostril. When you reach a complete exhalation, inhale through your right nostril. At your full inhalation, switch from your index finger to cover the right nostril with your thumb and exhale through your left nostril. Continue this sequence:

> Inhale left, exhale right
> Inhale right, exhale left
> Inhale left, exhale right

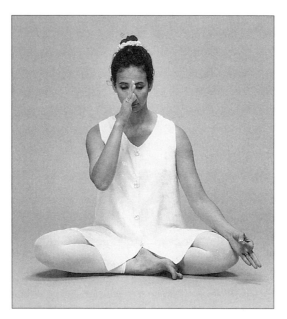

Alternate Nostril Breathing

Breathe conscious long, deep breaths. Keep your breath smooth without straining. You can concentrate on the sound of your breath or the mantra *Sat* on the inhale and *Naam* on the exhale. Meditate in this manner for 3–31 minutes.

Benefits Yogic science applies different attributes to left and right nostril breathing. Breathing through the left nostril (associated with the right brain) is described as cooling and promotes a relaxed, receptive attitude. Breathing through the right nostril (associated with the left brain) encourages a warmer and more energized state. Alternate nostril breathing is a basic and beautiful way to bring balance to the hemispheres of your brain. It is a powerful tonic to your nervous and glandular system, and is highly recommended for practice throughout your life. Mastering this meditation is said to help you maintain your sense of balance and spirit through the hormonal changes experienced during perimenopause, monthly menstruation, and menopause.

Grace of God Meditation

Yogi Bhajan says of this meditation: "Grace of God meditation will give you self-effectiveness. It is designed that way. Any woman who does it will find grace in her behavior. It may take a little time, but the results will be positive."

Grace of God is a two-part meditation. You can practice each part separately, but for best results, practice the meditation as given. Lie on your back. Relax your face and body, close your eyes, and rest your arms by your side with your palms facing upward. Inhale deeply and suspend your breath in your body. As you hold the breath in, mentally repeat "I am Grace of God" ten times. Exhale, hold your breath out, and mentally repeat the affirmation again ten times. Continue this sequence for five complete breaths. You will have repeated the affirmation one hundred times.

After you complete the above sequence, relax your breath and keep your eyes closed. Sit up in Easy Pose. Rest your right hand in Gyan Mudra (index finger and thumb meeting to form a circle) on your right knee with your elbow straight. Hold your left hand up by your left shoulder with your palm facing away from you and your fingers extended upward (as if you are taking an oath). Keep your breath relaxed. Bend one finger at a time, keeping the other fingers extended, as you repeat the affirmation aloud "I am Grace of God" five times with each finger. While repeating the affirmation, meditate on the corresponding energy of each finger (as shown on page 86). When you complete all five repetitions, lower your hand and relax for a few minutes.

Benefits This meditation is easy to do and has a powerful effect on your mind and body. The breath sequence breaks stressful breath patterns. When you are under stress, you often unconsciously exaggerate your inhalation or exhalation, which upsets your energy balance. If you are over-inhaling, you can feel out of breath, never relaxed. If you are overexhaling, you can feel exhausted and lacking in energy and presence. This breath sequence breaks that pattern. Combining this breath with the affirmation and confirmation in the second part affects your totality. This meditation can cut through feelings of insecurity and isolation, and assist you in affirming your infinite identity. It can help you develop the self-confidence you need to fulfill your destiny. Grace can be described as the total inner beauty and strength of each woman, the radiant strength that penetrates through even the most challenging situations.

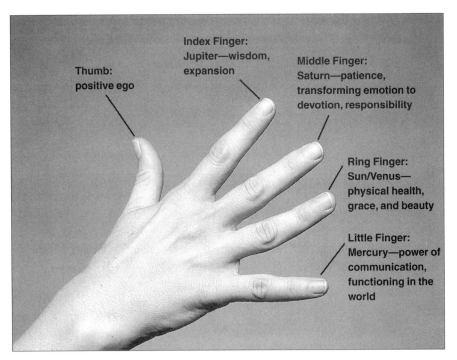

Hand illustrating qualities represented by each finger

Healing PMS

The goal of the awakened woman is to be sensitive to her body during all her cycles and transitions. As a matter of fact, the more yoga, exercise, meditation, and self-awareness a woman practices, the more deeply she will feel these sensations within her body. A practicing yogini can sense ovulation, hormonal changes, and imbalances in her reproductive system.

PMS is different from the normal sensations of a menstrual period. In the second 2 weeks of her cycle, a woman with PMS may feel unusually irritable, depressed, and fatigued. She may experience abdominal bloating, swollen hands and feet, breast tenderness, and headaches. It may be harder for her to be a good parent or to act "normal" toward her partner or coworkers.

Keep in mind that some degree of premenstrual symptoms is normal in all women. A healthy lifestyle, including yoga, meditation and relaxation, social activity, and proper diet, balances the menstrual cycles of most women. Realize, too, that it is natural to feel the shifting of hormones in your body.

Awareness of your hormones and your ability to flow with them is a goal of yoga for women. If PMS interferes with your behavior to the extent that you are unable to function, your menstrual cycle is most likely unbalanced.

Imbalances in body, mind, and spirit are viewed holistically in yoga. Healing PMS from this perspective means looking closely at three elements: how you are eating, how you are moving, and how you are thinking. A woman with PMS should eat a light diet of only fresh foods. Eliminate processed food completely for as long as you feel comfortable to cleanse the system and give your digestion a rest. Exercise each day until you sweat, except for the days you are menstruating. Sweating indicates that you have exercised enough to affect your glandular system. If you don't currently exercise, start with a short walk to build your strength. Specific yoga exercises can also help return your cycle to a balanced state; these are outlined further on in this section.

Finally, to deal with how you think, evaluate the stress in your life, especially your level of anger and frustration. The present cultural norms do not accept a woman in her totality: youth, middle age, and seniority. It is impossible for women to live up to the standards to which the media hold them. Over time these unreasonable expectations can create anger, frustration, and depression. In addition, traumas from the past, especially negative or violent sexual encounters, can have a profound impact on a woman's sense of well-being. Feelings of resentment and helplessness can become chronic. This type of chronic anger can negatively and directly affect a woman's menstrual cycle, hormonal balance, and ovaries.

The yogini finds a way to process her feelings through *devotion* as opposed to *commotion* and tantrums. Many women heal PMS through a variety of methods, including yoga and meditation, diet, exercise, Chinese and other herbal therapies, and progesterone, calcium, and magnesium homeopathy—in fact, any combination of therapeutic techniques. Use the power of commitment and break through your confusion and imbalance by adopting a rigorous meditation practice. Locate a knowledgeable and experienced Kundalini Yoga teacher and join a class. If you can attend a woman's meditation or support group, the support you receive can help your practice gain momentum.

Be methodical and intelligent with each healing technique and don't give up. Work with people you trust. Meditate and pray daily for your healing. In addition, socialize with women to create sisterhood and support, and be committed to freeing yourself from repressed anger and resentment. Motivate yourself toward actions that elevate and heal you. By making these efforts on your own behalf, you will go far in the process of healing. You will also be working in partnership with your doctor to achieve the best possible results using the least invasive medications and methods.

CRITERIA FOR PMS

1. The presence by self-report of at least one of the following somatic *and* behavioral symptoms during the 5 days before menses in each of the three previous menstrual cycles:

Behavioral	Somatic
Depression	Breast tenderness
Angry outbursts	Abdominal bloating
Irritability	Headache
Anxiety	Swelling
Confusion	
Social withdrawal	

2. Relief of the above symptoms within 4 days of your period with no return of the symptoms until day 12 of your menstrual cycle.

3. Symptoms occur in the absence of any medicines.

4. Symptoms repeat for two cycles in a row.

5. Identifiable dysfunction in social or economic performance by one of the following criteria:

> Marital or relationship discord confirmed by partner
> Difficulties in parenting
> Poor work or school performance (attendance/tardiness)
> Increased social isolation
> Legal difficulties
> Suicidal thoughts
> Seeking medical attention for somatic symptoms

The following exercises are recommended as preventative yoga prescriptions for PMS. These exercises are to be done daily, throughout the month, except when you have your period. During the days of peak flow, follow the basic guidelines for exercises, diet, and rest. The first three exercises can be done individually or as a set.

Plough Pose—Back Massage

Lie flat on your back. Lift your legs over your head, supporting your back, and stretch until your toes touch the floor over your head. Do not roll onto your neck. If your toes cannot reach the floor, let your legs stay parallel to the floor. After you stretch for a few seconds (do not hold the posture, just feel the stretch briefly), gently roll out of the stretch and lie flat on your back again. Continue this rolling motion for 2–3 minutes. To end, relax on your back for a few minutes.

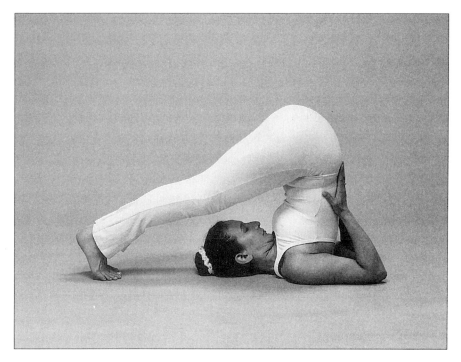

Plough Pose

Benefits This exercise stretches out your back and legs. It stimulates digestion, elimination, and the release of tension in the entire back, including the reproductive organs.

Frog Pose—for Circulation, Digestion, and the Glandular System

Squat with your knees apart and your heels off the floor, touching each other. Place your hands on the floor between your knees for balance. Inhale as you straighten your legs and raise your buttocks up, looking at your knees. Keep your hands on the floor and your heels off the floor. Exhale as you squat down. Repeat this sequence for 1–3 minutes.

If you cannot touch the floor while you straighten your legs, take time to develop flexibility with some spine and leg flexibility exercises. Go at a steady pace, keep up, and do your best.

Benefits Frog Pose can improve sexual function and energy and helps stretch the life nerve (the sciatic nerve complex). This exercise increases the circulation of your blood and glandular system throughout the body, including circulation to your breasts. See also Life-Nerve Stretch in Chapter 10.

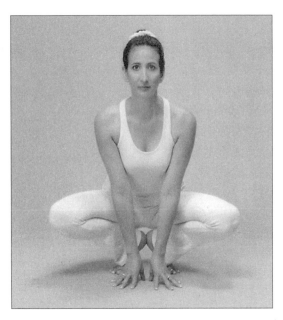

Frog Pose in squat position

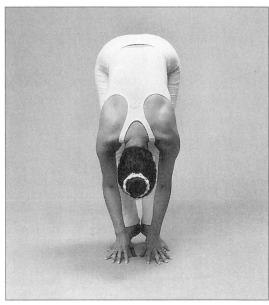

Frog Pose in stretched position

Knees-to-Chest Pose

Lying on your back, draw your knees toward your chest and wrap your arms around your legs, holding on to your shins. Relax your head and neck. Breathe in a relaxed, normal breathing pattern, or do Long, Deep Breathing. If you feel too much tension in your knees, hold your legs by the back of your thighs instead of by your shins.

Benefits This posture provides a gentle stretch for your lower back and massages your ovaries and reproductive organs. Relax in this posture anytime you want to relax your back, relieve tension in your ovaries, or relax your mind. Practice this posture as often as you wish to begin tuning into your feminine body and healing your menstrual discomfort or PMS symptoms.

Lower-Back Stretch—Massage for Ovaries and Proper Menstruation

Extend your right leg straight out in front of you. Place your left foot on the top of your right thigh. Reach behind your back and interlace your fingers. Lean forward from the hip area and stretch, reaching your nose toward your

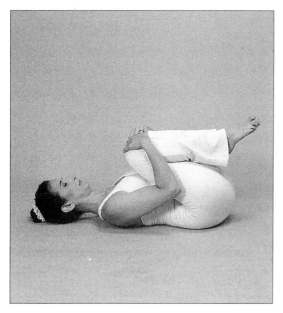

Knees-to-Chest Pose for lower-back relaxation

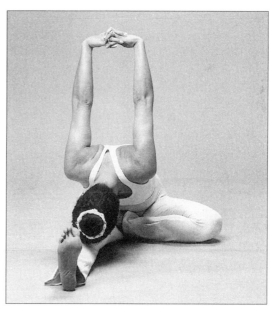

Lower-Back Stretch

right knee while stretching your arms up behind you. Stretch the arms as high as possible. Do not push too hard; build up flexibility for a few seconds at first without feeling tension in your neck or knees. Hold this posture with Long, Deep Breathing for a maximum of 1–2 minutes. To end, inhale and hold the breath briefly, exhale, and relax.

Benefits This exercise is good for the ovaries and promotes proper menstruation. It is also good for releasing excess gas from the digestive system. Excess gas and poor elimination can aggravate PMS. Do not push too hard; build up flexibility without creating tension in your neck or knees. Try holding for a few seconds to start, and build up your time as your strength and flexibility increase.

Nine Yoga Exercises to Release Premenstrual Tension

These nine exercises release tension and increase strength. You will find some of these exercises easier to do than others, so build up your strength and flexibility slowly. For the best results, do all nine exercises as a set. However, if this set is more than you can do, try some of the more gentle yoga exercises or walk 30 minutes daily and try the breath meditation at the end of the series.

Exercise 1, a meditation for deep relaxation, helps balance hormones. Exercises 2 and 3 can relieve tension in your ovaries. Exercises 4 and 5 stimulate the circulation and energy in your digestive system and navel point (a yogic area very important to balance and vitality), which can increase the circulation of your glandular secretions and work directly on your hormones. Exercise 6 stimulates blood circulation in your ovaries and your head. Exercise 7 can help reduce recurrent headaches. Exercise 8 helps to release mental tension. This exercise set can be challenging and rigorous and will give you the benefits of strong exercise. If you experience chronic tension or PMS, it is recommended that you practice this set daily for 40 days (except during the days of menstruation).

1. **Leg Extension.** Begin by sitting on your heels. Extend your left leg straight behind you and bend forward, touching your forehead to the floor. Place your arms along your sides with your palms facing upward. Relax in this posture for up to 3 minutes. To end, inhale and

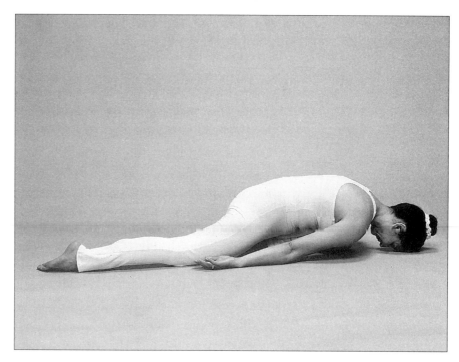

Leg Extension

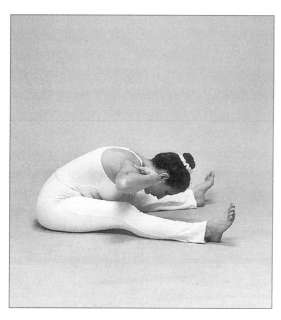

Forward Stretch

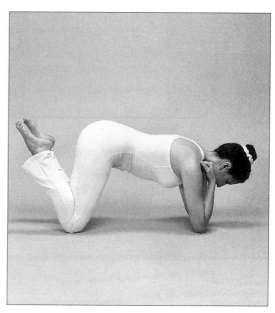

Hands-and-Knees Walk

hold the breath briefly, exhale, and relax. Release the posture by using your hands to help you sit up as you draw your left leg forward, sitting on your heels again. Rest a moment and switch legs, holding the posture with the right leg stretched behind you for 3 minutes.

2. *Throat Massage.* Begin by sitting on your heels. Massage your throat from your collarbone to under your chin for 2 minutes. Then massage your ears and your ear lobes with the palms of your hands. Move your palms up and down, as well as in circles. Continue for 2–3 minutes. This massage works on pressure points and meridian points that relate to your ovaries.

3. *Spinal Twist.* While sitting on your heels, clasp your hands behind you at the small of your back, interlacing your fingers, then exhale and slowly twist to your right. Continue breathing and twisting your spine slowly for up to 3 minutes. To end, inhale and face forward, then exhale and feel energy going into the center of your spine.

4. *Forward Stretch.* Begin this exercise by lying flat on your back on the floor. Grasp your shoulders with your thumbs in back and your fingers in front. Let your elbows relax on the floor. Spread your legs as wide as possible. Meditate and concentrate on all your muscles and, as slowly as possible, muscle by muscle, keeping your abdominal muscles tight, lift the body forward until you are sitting all the way up and bending forward until your nose touches the ground. Hold the stretch, leaning forward with your legs spread apart for up to 3 minutes. To end, take a deep breath, sit up, and relax.

5. *Nose-to-Knee Stretch.* Start this exercise the same way that you did Exercise 4, but this time bring your nose to your left knee and hold for up to 1 minute. Then inhale and exhale three times and lie back down on the floor. Repeat the exercise, this time bringing your nose to your right knee. To end, inhale and exhale three times, then relax.

6. *Hands-and-Knees Walk.* Begin this exercise by crouching on your hands and knees. Raise your forearms so your upper body is resting on your elbows. Raise your lower legs off the floor. You are now balancing on your hands and knees. Raise your head and begin to walk!

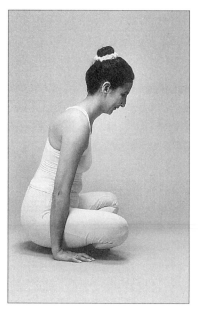

Cross-Legged Walk

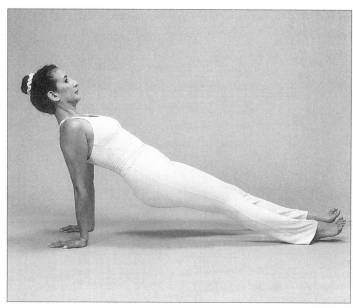

Hands-and-Heels Walk

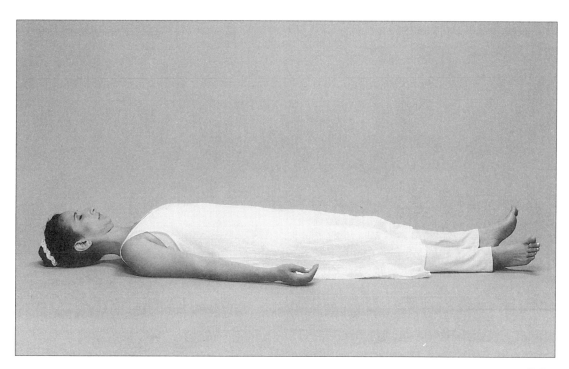

Relax

Keep your feet pressed as close to your buttocks as possible while you try walking. Continue for up to 3 minutes, then relax on your back.

7. ***Cross-Legged Walk.*** Sit in Easy Pose (legs crossed with a straight spine). Put your hands on the floor beside you and try to scoot along the floor by bending forward and lifting your lower body off the floor. Continue for up to 3 minutes. To end, uncross your legs and relax.

8. ***Hands-and-Heels Walk.*** Begin this exercise by sitting straight with your legs stretched out in front of you. Put your hands on the floor in back of you. Lift your buttocks off the floor, without bending your knees, and walk on your heels and your hands (you can bend your waist slightly). Continue for up to 3 minutes. To end, release the posture and relax.

9. ***Relax.*** Hold Corpse Pose for 15 minutes. Lie flat on your back and relax deeply.

The Benefits of This Exercise Set

Many of the painful symptoms experienced during menstruation can result from tension building up in your body and, more specifically, in your ovaries. Once a month during ovulation, your ovaries go through a very slow contraction or lifting motion, which can be aggravated by tension. Exercising frequently can help relieve this problem and reduce your pain by releasing tension and balancing your glandular system.

DR.'S NOTES

PMS

PMS is not a product of modern society. Hippocrates recognized the symptoms of premenstrual syndrome, but it wasn't until 1931 that Dr. R. T. Frank discovered that PMS was a hormonal condition. We now know that approximately 5 out of 100 women experience this problem. In the last sixty years great progress has been made in understanding PMS better, but much about it remains a mystery.

While we know that women who suffer from PMS often feel out of control, scientifically, we don't know why. In fact, women with and without PMS have the same psychological scores using standard personality tests and the same results using biochemical markers.

PMS manifests in at least four different ways: cravings, bloating, anxiety, and depression. Many possibilities have been suggested to explain its occurrence, including the fact that changing levels of brain opiates, the powerful hormones that affect mood and behavior, can change the experience of your menstrual cycle.

The first week after you ovulate, brain opiate levels are high and may cause the binge eating that is often associated with PMS. During the second week after ovulation, the last week of your menstrual cycle, blood levels of the brain opiate beta-endorphin fall rapidly. These levels are even lower if you have PMS. This causes a kind of opiate withdrawal that may lead to the irritability, anxiety, tension, and even aggression some women describe. Exercise helps to balance brain opiates and may even elevate them. That is why many women experiencing PMS benefit from vigorous exercise. The yoga set we have suggested in this section is rigorous and will address this problem directly.

Other brain hormones, such as serotonin, GABA, 5-HT, and even adrenaline, may play a role in producing PMS symptoms. Although the exact role they play is still not certain, meditation, relaxation, and stress management often prove beneficial because they lower adrenaline and cortisol, and may affect brain hormone levels as well.

Vitamin and mineral deficiencies may also play a role in PMS. Some doctors believe that PMS is a result of vitamin B_6 deficiency. Good food sources of B_6 include soybeans, whole wheat, legumes, green leafy vegetables, bananas, and figs. Although the Recommended Daily Intake (RDI) for B_6 is 6 mg daily, women are being instructed to take 100–200 mg daily. Some women will feel better with these dosages, but apparently not better than women treated with placebo. If you are taking higher dosages of B_6 and notice tingling or numbness in your hands or feet, notify your doctor and stop taking it. These higher levels may cause damage to your nerve endings.

Other studies suggest that low levels of magnesium and calcium lead to PMS symptoms. Daily dosages of 100–400 mg of magnesium and 500–1,000 mg of calcium are recommended for all women, especially those who suffer from PMS. In one study, 73 percent of women taking calcium reported global improvement of their symptoms, as compared with 15 percent who took a placebo. It may take up to 3 months for the full benefits of calcium intake to take effect. As you can see, many forms of treatment can work for many women, but none works for all.

Some women who think they have PMS are actually clinically depressed. Depression usually lasts all month long, whereas PMS occurs only in the last half of your cycle. If your symptoms are so strong for two weeks in a row, or all month long that you feel sad or lack the motivation and the vitality you know are possible for you, talk with your doctor or mental health provider. Depression is treatable.

Medical treatment options for PMS, however, are still limited. If PMS is severe and a woman does not respond to natural remedies such as diet, lifestyle, and therapeutic meditation, drug therapies such as selective serotonin reuptake inhibitors (SSRIs), including Prozac and Zoloft, are being tried. Because of their many possible side effects, drugs such as Prozac should be considered as a path of treatment only after serious discussion with your physician and therapist.

Beware of fad "PMS diets," especially those that do not provide you with balanced nutrition. By contrast, healthy whole foods and certain herbs contain many healing qualities and vast storehouses of phytochemicals helpful to women with PMS. In general, make every effort to reduce the intake of salt, caffeine, refined sugars, and refined carbohydrates, especially during the second half of your cycle. For example, try couscous, kasha, or unrefined rice instead of white pasta; use lemon instead of salt; and follow the dietary recommendations for healthy menstruation found earlier in this chapter.

One herb worthy of note is chasteberry, also known as vitex. It is just beginning to be appreciated in the United States, but it has been used for menstrual problems since ancient Roman times and is recommended by the Commission E, Germany's herbal regulatory body for the treatment of PMS. Try 175–225 mg daily in tablets or capsules, or 2 milliliters daily in liquid extract. Licorice root (*Glycerrhiza glabra*) has become a popular remedy for PMS, but be careful: Higher dosages of licorice can lead to high blood pressure and elevated levels of potassium. Patients with kidney disease or glaucoma should avoid it.

FOODS FOR PMS

Certain foods are particularly good for a woman with PMS. Ginger and chamomile teas are beverages of choice and may relieve menstrual cramps. Before menstruation begins, eat a diet high in fiber. Remember, poor elimination adds stress during the menstrual cycle. Before, during, and 4–5 days after your period, take 1–3 teaspoons of sesame oil daily. According to the science of yoga, this can help prevent any feeling of weakness during menstruation. While menstruating, eat a light diet so you can digest your food easily. Following menstruation, eat a high-fiber diet for 5–7 days.

PMS Tea—A Tea for Energy and Youth

- 1 teaspoon ground cardamom
- 1 heaping tablespoon basil
- 1 cup water

Combine ingredients and boil for 20 minutes, adding more water if necessary. Add maple syrup or molasses for a sweetener. Make certain the tea is hot. Sip with a tablespoon. Start with a cup in the morning and one at 4:00 P.M. If it is helpful, additional cups can be taken at noon and at 8:00 P.M.

YOGA AT HOME: MENSTRUATION

Healing Your Cycle

Try the Cold Water Therapy (see Chapter 11), but not during menstruation, and/or self-massage. Massage your ovaries (the area around your belly button, hips, and pubic bone) every morning.

1. Tune in.

2. Alternate Nostril Breathing for 7–11 minutes. Alternate Nostril Breathing will help stimulate your hypothalamus and balance your hormonal structure, moods, and brain hemispheres.

3. Spinal Flex and Spinal Twist to warm up your spine and massage the ovaries.

4. Do one or all of the following yoga postures with a few minutes' rest between postures.
   - Half-Wheel Pose
   - Tiger Stretch
   - Cobra Pose
   - Bow Pose
   - Leg Lifts

5. Breath meditation to regulate your menstrual cycle.

6. Relax.

7. Choose two diet and lifestyle suggestions and incorporate them into your life.

Healing PMS

Beginner's Daily Practice

1. Tune in.

2. Breath of Fire or Long, Deep Breathing twenty-six times, or for 1–3 minutes.

3. Spinal Flex and Spinal Twist exercises for ovarian massage and releasing tension.

4. Knees-to-Chest Pose to relax your lower back.

5. Forward Stretch or Lower-Back Stretch.

6. Alternate Nostril Breathing for 3–11 minutes.

7. Relax for 11 minutes.

8. Grace of God Meditation—twice daily. This meditation can be done at any time during the day or before bed.

9. Walk for 15–30 minutes daily.

Advanced Daily Practice

1. Tune in.

2. Breath of Fire or Long, Deep Breathing for 3 minutes.

3. Yoga exercise set to release premenstrual tension (page 92).

4. Deep relaxation for 11 minutes.

5. Alternate Nostril Breathing for 11–31 minutes.

6. Walk 1–5 miles daily.

7. Grace of God Meditation.

For extreme PMS that is interfering with your functioning, see your doctor and pursue alternative therapies that suit you. The Alternate Nostril Breathing for 31 minutes is a rigorous and effective practice. Build up to that time, starting with 11 minutes, if you need to. Practice these recommendations as early in the day as you can to avoid any sleep disturbances, which can occur if you exercise too late in the day.

QUESTIONS FOR FURTHER GROWTH

- What is your present attitude toward your menstrual period? Observe the first thought you have when you realize you are getting your period. Is it negative, positive, or neutral?

- Map your menstrual cycle. Evaluate your cycle. Is it a 28-day cycle? Are your periods painful, or is the cramping extensive? What yoga, meditation, and lifestyle suggestions from this chapter can you integrate into your life?

- Do you respect the physical, mental, and spiritual significance of your menstrual cycle?

- How has having PMS affected your life? Journal the history of your difficulties, including the therapies you have tried and their results. Evaluate your present state of health regarding PMS.

- Do you experience continuous or frequent states of anger and resentment that make you feel out of control?

- Can you forgive those around you and yourself for the past and for any important issues?

- What would be your next step in healing PMS? Methodically plan and realistically integrate suggested lifestyle changes and locate doctors and health practitioners whom you trust to assist you.

6

Sexuality, Intimacy, and Pleasure— The Yogini Way

The sexual relationship is such an important and valued part of God's design that in the spiritual world it is called "the throne of creativity."

—YOGI BHAJAN

This earth plane is a playground for the senses. Filling your home with scented flowers, pillows and fabrics of beauty, and foods that consciously stimulate your senses is healing, uplifting, and part of the yogini life. The yogini believes that sensual pleasures are God's gift to us and that they can be in harmony with our spiritual path and social responsibilities. According to the teachings of an ancient text, the *Kama Sutra,* one's sensuality is supposed to be in balance with *Dharma,* one's spiritual path. One can enjoy the *Kama*—the pleasures of life and the sensuality of love and marriage—while walking the path of *Dharma*—spiritual awareness. And one can follow *Artha*—earning a righteous living and amassing wealth for one's family and community—while experiencing both Dharma and Kama. In the yogini's life, all three—Artha, Dharma, and Kama—are designed to be in harmony.

When you are living in this harmony, you are fully participating in life and worldly events, while remaining aware of life's deeper meaning and larger perspective. The regular practice of Kundalini Yoga is designed to help you achieve this precious harmony between the material world and the spirit. For women, this is good news! Living in the world has historically been considered a deterrent to spiritual growth, and in some cultures, women are denied full access to their sexuality. The path of Kundalini Yoga is one that embraces all aspects of living in the world, including intimate relationships and sex.

Sexuality, from the perspective of Kundalini Yoga and the teachings of Yogi Bhajan, can be a powerfully spiritual, loving experience that can further spiritual growth and increase the depth of your loving relationship. However, when sexuality is divorced from spirit, the result is tragic. Sex and sexuality in Western culture continue to be viewed in the narrowest sense of their meanings. As a culture we have become unconscious of the primal power and broader meaning of sexual energy. It is precisely because of its great power that sex and sexuality are often misunderstood, abused, and used for inappropriate purposes. Sex is used to sell products, as a hook to market goods and people, to subjugate, to abuse, and to gain power. Young people learn about sex only in the context of anatomy, spreading disease, or becoming pregnant, often without the information on the profound effect sex has on the mind, body, and soul. As people grow older, sex continues to be viewed as an isolated act, rather than as an integrated facet of a whole person. Our common Western perspective does not set the foundation for a healthy sexual relationship. Perhaps this is why 43 percent of women and 31 percent of men in the United States say they experience sexual dysfunction!

By contrast, the yogini approaches her sexual energy with a sacred attitude. Sexuality is viewed as the primal force of energy within each human being. Your sexual energy and urges are in fact a powerful creative energy that can be refined to develop satisfying sexual relationships or that can be transformed into energy for other creative and spiritual endeavors.

The yogis describe sexual energy in several different ways. It is an "urge to merge" with another person, the energy of two people longing to be one. The sacred act of sex can be the fulfillment of a happy and cozy relationship. Sexual energy is also the seed of creativity. It is the twinkle of the child in the eye of the mother and father. It is the spark of creativity for the artist, the musician, and the inspired poet. The power of sex can be harnessed and transformed so it becomes available for creativity, the soul's expression in the material world as a divine manifestation. Sexuality is the life energy that is beyond time or space. Using this primal power, the yogini can experience a union between herself and another, or between herself and her creator.

The guidance and suggestions here are practical and down to earth. If you develop your awareness and sensitivity, you can contain and direct this powerful energy in ways that are fulfilling and true for you. It is *vital* that you understand the power of your sexuality, presentation, and presence as a woman. You hold the power to elevate all with just a smile or a glance. When you elevate yourself with self-love, you elevate all those around you.

The Yoga of Sex

In its basic nature, sexuality is the most powerful form of energy, the very energy of creation: Sex creates life! Sexual energy is actually creative energy focused toward reproduction. This energy is available at all times. Through the practice of Kundalini Yoga, you can harness your sexual energy and transform it for healing, spiritual development, and creativity. Following are some yogini sex "basics."

Keep Your Body Healthy

Your body is your temple. Take care of it as best you can, whatever your limitations, and your reward will be increased vitality and attractiveness. Daily exercise and the practicing of yoga postures are helpful in maintaining a healthy glandular system and a strong physical projection. Your glands, especially the thyroid, pituitary, and pineal glands, regulate weight and are responsible for the sexual response. Regular practice of Kundalini Yoga helps keep your glandular system operating at peak efficiency.

Develop a Clear, Relaxed, and Meditative Mind

When you have the ability to concentrate and be present in your life, your self-awareness is great. You are less distracted and better able to participate in the moment. Don't let an overactive and emotional mind prevent you from enjoying your sex life! Meditation can teach you to quiet your mind, which is especially important during sex.

Bring Sacredness into Your Daily Life

Sex expresses the attraction of the opposites, male and female, and represents the ultimate union. View sexuality, then, as a sacred act, an act of ultimate intimacy and expressed love. If you become calm and relaxed, you can become sensitive to your needs and the needs of your partner. Express yourself kindly, openly, and without fear. Communicate with your partner to develop honesty and trust. The Venus Kriyas—Yoga for Couples—are included in this chapter to help you deepen both your trust in and attraction for your sexual partner.

Maintain an Enlightened View of Sexuality

Sex begins in your head! The first signal of sexual stimulation comes from your brain, specifically, the yogis believe, your pituitary gland. Once stimulated, the secretions of your glands—the hormonal elixirs—flow throughout your body to signal desire, readiness, and a host of complex thoughts and sensations that can lead to a powerful sexual union.

Your glandular system is stimulated by all of your senses. When your senses are enlivened, your thoughts follow, and a powerful feedback loop is created. The sense of sight is the most powerful stimulus of sexual feelings. The next most powerful is sound; the third, touch; and the fourth, smell. You are also stimulated by the fragrance of your partner; your sensitive hormonal system can pick up the scent of a man on a subtle, subconscious level. (These sensitivities are the basis for fragrances, perfumes, aphrodisiacs, lingerie, and many other sexual stimulants.)

The knowledge of the power of the senses and the environment in sexual stimulation enables yogis to choose surroundings appropriate to the senses they want to stimulate. Your senses can be a gateway to enlightenment or a pathway to self-destruction. The yogini chooses her environment to represent her highest potential, and her sexuality is a conscious, powerful expression of love and union.

Create True Intimacy

Trusting relationships create the intimacy necessary for a healthy, enjoyable sexual relationship. Some women, however, may misunderstand intimacy and see it as the result, not the precursor, of a sexual act. Especially in young women—although present in women of all ages who are awakening to their sexuality—the sexual drive is so strong that it can dominate their thinking and sensations. Without understanding the reality of sex and love, many women feel that having sex will bring them love, intimacy, and fulfillment. It is for this reason that many women often find their sexual encounters continually disappointing and often psychologically damaging. A clear understanding of sexuality is a must for all women; a lack of understanding of the power of sexuality is an invitation to abuse, confusion, exploitation, and unhappiness. It is vital for a woman to learn how to transform her powerful sexual urge and energy into devotion to her spiritual essence and creativity.

Another issue affecting women's sexuality is exploitation by advertising and the media. The blatant sexual orientation of the media hooks both women and men into a game of sexual teasing. This barrage of "hooking" keeps people caught in the negative aspects of their lower chakras—the need for security, the confusion of "sex as love," and the drive to obtain power over others. In the philosophy of yoga, intimacy can flourish in a relationship only when both partners are operating primarily from the higher chakras by opening their hearts and becoming aware of the divine spirit within each other. The yogini doesn't get hooked into her momentary desires in this illusory world. Her goal is to live a balanced life that will allow the energies of all the chakras to interact and through this interaction balance her human and divine qualities. This balance is the union the yogini seeks.

Be Kind in Your Attitude Toward Sex

There are many times in a woman's life when sex is difficult, impossible, and inappropriate. Couples educated in the art of love understand the difference between sex and love. As you age, your energy naturally moves more into your higher chakras, and sexuality, although enjoyable, is not the focus of life. At this stage, intimacy can be at its height.

While in most situations it is best to be very clear and direct when communicating with your partner, feedback regarding sexual satisfaction can be a sensitive topic. When discussing sex, it is best to avoid being confrontational. Be kind and considerate and discuss sex when you are calm. Intercourse is not the time for discourse!

Where, When, and How Often

Sex is a conscious act that should energize the couple, nurture the family, and enrich the home. Avoid engaging in sexual activities on a full stomach, when you are angry or upset, or when you are overly tired; it's not good for you, and it's not good for your relationship. If you are tired but want to participate, you can take a moment to increase your energy with some stretching and Breath of Fire. These will help you concentrate on your pleasurable sensations and enjoy yourself. Alternatively, if the time is not right, enjoy the closeness of each other and wait for a more optimal time.

Do not have sex if you are insecure or fearful about the environment or the relationship. Each act of sexual intercourse deeply imprints itself upon a woman. You are the receiver of the seed, and even though the act of sex may end, it remains in your psyche as an imprint, like an image imprinted on the film of a camera. The male gives the seed to the woman, and when intercourse is over, he does not carry as deep an imprint on his psyche. Many women have difficulty healing after negative sexual experiences because their pain becomes so deeply rooted. In these situations therapy can be helpful, and Kirtan Kriya (the chanting meditation in Chapter 4), which cleanses the woman's aura and subconscious of past sexual experiences, can also be of benefit.

The frequency of sexual activity is also discussed in Kundalini Yoga. One sexual union per month is generally recommended in order to keep your energy contained and creative. This is far from what most couples consider "normal" in the West. In order to fairly evaluate this teaching, consider the sacredness of sex, the gathering of the energy so that the sexual encounter is fully satisfying and mutual, and the powerful effects of the union. Busy couples use so much of their energy and still feel guilty if they don't have sex. Women care for children and work, men work and feel the stress of providing, and still spouses complain that they are not sexually available! A couple needs to work together, communicate, and understand the reality and power of their sexual energy in relation to the energy they need to keep their lives going smoothly. If they maintain a healthy reverence and respect for each other and the roles they play in their family, they can enjoy a fulfilling sex life without guilt or pressure. Let go of your expectations and investigate the joys of having a spiritual sexual relationship. These yogic guidelines may be factored into consideration, without guilt or judgment of oneself or one's partner.

The Yogic Sexual Experience

Sexual pleasure is an art and a science. It is an open conversation between lovers and a topic of ongoing study. For the yogin and the yogini, sexuality can be a powerful yogic practice as well as an avenue of fulfillment and pleasure. Says Yogi Bhajan: "In physical intercourse, everything should be at its optimum: time, space, body's action, nerves, desires, thought, imagination, and energy. You cohabit in such a way that you both lose your individual sense of identity . . . as the sexual union progresses, both lovers reach a stage of extreme relaxation and totally merge as a unity of combined polarity. This is an experience of ecstasy. This is what ideally happens in sexual life. Both partners melt into one another and never know what is going on, where they are, who they are, or what happened. This experience is beyond time and space."

Please note that same-sex partners can also find much of this information useful. For further discussions regarding same-sex intimacy, please refer to the book *Sacred Sexual Bliss* by Dr. Sat Kaur Khalsa.

Extended Foreplay

Sex should begin 72 hours before intercourse. This is usually the most exciting news most women hear when they learn the yogini way of sexuality! A woman takes time and enjoys the game of warming up and anticipating being with her lover. This game involves more than scheduling sex; it is literally 72 hours of foreplay! Start with sexy talk, gestures, and glances. You can do Kundalini Yoga (together or alone) to energize your physical body, chakras, and Subtle Anatomy so you feel balanced, secure, and energized. Try applying sandalwood-scented oil to your inner thighs, as this is said to increase desire. You can have lots of fun with this kind of foreplay. You will know when the time comes to take it to the bedroom.

If you're worried that your partner might not want to participate in extended foreplay, don't; it won't be hard to convince him to play this game if you are open and honest. Communicate that you want to have the best sex ever and that you would like to try this new yoga way of teasing and anticipating sex. You will be surprised how much fun, energy, and intimacy it can generate!

You can use your Moon Center locations (see Chapter 4 to review these) to enhance your sexual experience. The following Moon Centers should be stimulated before intercourse: the hairline on your forehead, your lips, your ears and the back of your neck, your breast area, your navel point area (or belly and lower back), and your thighs.

In addition to these Moon Centers, your partner can massage your body as follows: Have your partner massage your breasts patiently. Your breasts need this massage to prepare them so the nipples can be touched and stimulated. This is a requirement for women during foreplay.

After your breasts have been massaged so that your nipples can be touched and kissed, have your partner massage and kiss your neck and lips. Kissing on the lips stimulates many other parts of your body. From here, have him touch your cheeks, the hairline around your face (your arc line or halo), and then your ears. Your ears are a microcosm of your entire body (in some traditions, the earlobes are considered just as sensitive as the nipples). From these two areas, the nipples and the earlobes, your energy will open downward, toward your genitals. Have him massage your inner thighs next, as your sexual energy rises and you begin opening up for intercourse. After stimulating your inner thighs, your partner can massage your calves. Then you are ready to open up to his massage of your clitoris or vagina.

This methodical massage, which is stimulating, relaxing, and helpful in readying you for intercourse, should take no less than 30 minutes to 1 hour. The massage follows the true movement of sexual energy, beginning at the pituitary gland and the upper areas of the body, and slowly moving downward through the chakras and toward the sexual organs. As the woman is massaged in this way, her aura grows from 7 to 9 feet!

As your partner is massaging and stimulating your Moon Centers, you can stimulate his erogenous centers. Massage his head, hair, and scalp, including his hairline and face. Then move downward to his buttocks, the inside of his thighs, his testicles, his penis, and his navel point and chest. You can intensify his orgasm by massaging his nipples during the orgasm. The opposing directions of the massage—woman from top down, and man from top up—are said to represent the merging of heaven and earth in the sexual union.

Your Moon Center changes every $2\frac{1}{2}$ days. You will feel extra sensitivity in the area corresponding to your Moon Center during foreplay and intercourse. If you and your partner are receptive to these massage techniques and sensitive to your Moon Centers, you can increase your sexual enjoyment and create a deeply intimate and energizing sexual relationship. Whichever Moon Center you are in at the time of the sexual encounter will be extra stimulating during foreplay. Some women have their partners help them get to know their Moon Centers in this manner. It is a fun game for the partner to find the "hot" Moon Center, even if you know it! Your Moon Centers are so sensitive that each one can act as an erogenous zone and through its stimulation may actually bring you to orgasm.

In general, men are sexually stimulated more easily than women and take less time to get ready for intercourse. As you slowly build toward sexual readiness, your partner should try to calm himself down. You can help him by supporting slow movements and maintaining a relaxed approach until you feel more heated and ready. Some of the more erotic areas for men include the nipples, inner thighs, chest, navel, and penis. Start massaging other areas, saving the latter for when you are more aroused.

Intercourse

Ideally, only after the woman is fully stimulated and her breasts are full and nipples erect should the man enter her. There are many positions for intercourse, and the comfort of the positions depends on the woman's anatomy and sensitivity. Intercourse for women, when fully prepared, should be pain-free and enjoyable. It is recommended that the male use a rotary motion to continually stimulate the nerves in the vagina.

Breath has both a stimulating and a calming effect during intercourse. It is said that if a woman is trying to conceive, she should practice the 1-minute breath before intercourse to deeply relax and enhance her receptivity. If you practice Long, Deep Breathing together with your partner before and during intercourse (see "Venus Kriyas" in this chapter), you intensify the blending of your auras as you move toward the union of your physical and subtle bodies, your minds, and your spirits.

If you breathe consciously and keep your attention on your upper bodies and faces, you can experience the power of sexual energy throughout your body and spine. Be open to experiencing sensation at your brow point, fingertips, and other parts of your body. As your aura mixes with your partner's, you can begin to feel limitless and unified. The energy you have stimulated together rises and enters the central channels of your spines. This merged energy is the basis for sexual ecstasy and the sacredness of the sexual union.

Orgasm

During intercourse, both man and woman work together to keep the energy merged as one. As mentioned before, all of a woman's Moon Centers can act as erogenous zones and bring her to orgasm. According to yogic teachings, it is important for a woman to have multiple "tidings" (orgasms) and for a male to have one. Without this culmination, the result can be frustrating and uncomfortable. There are many scientific studies and spiritual approaches that discuss the role of orgasm in the sexual act. If you are frustrated over not being able to achieve orgasm, you can seek help to evaluate both the physical and psychological aspects of your sexuality. Include your partner in your healing journey, if possible. Orgasm can be considered a point of realization for some yogis. It is an event when all time stops, boundaries disappear, and a Still Point and a sense of union can be experienced.

After Sex

During intercourse, the male and female auras mix. After climax is reached, it is important for the couple to relax together and experience their closeness. Often women are invigorated by sex, while men may be fatigued.

After intercourse, a woman should urinate and with cold water wash her face, armpits (to balance her parasympathetic nervous system), inner thighs, behind her ears, and her feet.

Foot Massage

Foot massage, as described in Chapter 11, has a primal healing quality within an intimate relationship. Trading foot massages can help you and your partner relax at the end of a busy day, stimulate healing and relaxation when your partner is in pain, and prepare you for more intimate encounters.

Sexual Chemistry   DR.'S NOTES

Lovers often speak of chemistry: something that they cannot quite touch, yet whose presence is undeniable. They are, in fact, correct. Although sex and sexuality can be quite physical, the origins of sexual chemistry are located far away from the pelvis or breasts. They are products of the mind. The scent of a lover, his smile or touch, sends impulses to the brain that eventually reach a brain center called the *nucleus accumbens*—the part of the brain associated with pleasure and the sexual responses we associate with romantic love. Through strong nerve links to sensory parts of the brain, to the frontal lobe, and to the hippocampus, where thoughts and memories are coordinated, the complex chemistry of sex is interpreted and translated.

Signals from our eyes entering through our optic nerves, from our nose entering through the olfactory nerves, and from our ears entering through the auditory nerves seep deeply into the brain, eventually finding their way to the hypothalamus and brain stem, where breathing, heart rate, sweating, blood vessels, and muscle tone are controlled. In a matter of moments, these inputs turn into physical signals that we perceive as sexually stimulating and arousing. Some sexual chemistry is due to *pheromones,* gaseous hormones that bind to receptors inside the nose within the *vomeronasal* organ. This is not the same gland that detects odors, but a highly specialized one in both men and women that enables the scent of these pheromones from women to stimulate men, and the virtually unscented pheromones of men to stimulate women.

Venus Kriyas—Partners' Yoga to Enhance an Intimate Relationship

The following Venus Kriyas—Seeing Yourself in Your Partner, Meditation to End an Argument, and Venus Life-Nerve Stretch—can have powerful effects on both you and your partner. These exercises combine posture, mudra, mantra, breathing, and meditation to create a strong energy between two people. This process blends the polarities of male and female and is designed to deepen love and divine consciousness. Do not use these practices for manipulation or ego gratification. Use them to elevate consciousness and to develop a deep connection with your partner.

To prepare for doing a Venus Kriya, follow these four steps:

1. Sit down opposite your partner and put your own hands together in prayer mudra (palms together with your hands in front of your chest). Tune in using the mantra *Ong Naamo Guroo Dayv Naamo.*

2. Next, chant the following mantra three times in a monotone. Chant one repetition of the entire mantra with each breath.

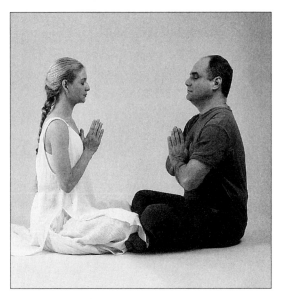

A couple tuning in

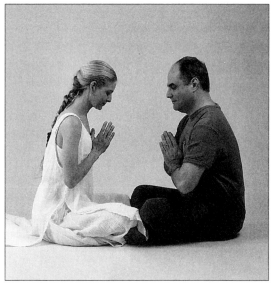

Bowing to begin

Aad Gurey Nameh (pronounced *ahd goo-ray nahmay*),
Jugad Gurey Nameh (pronounced *yoo-gahd goo-ray nah-may*),
Sat Gurey Nameh (pronounced *saht goo-ray nah-may*),
Siree Guroo Dayvay Nameh (pronounced *see-ree goo-roo day-vay nah-may*).

This mantra means:

I bow to the primal wisdom,
I bow to the wisdom of all the ages,
I bow to the truest Wisdom,
I bow to the great universal Wisdom.

3. With your hands still together, look into the eyes of your partner and project love and divine light—any loving thought or positive affirmation,

4. Bow your head in recognition of the divine consciousness in each other.

5. When you complete the Venus Kriya or meditation, stretch up, raising your hands above your head, and twist from side to side. Bring your hands together down in front of you again, look into the eyes of your partner, and say, "Thank you. *Sat Naam*."

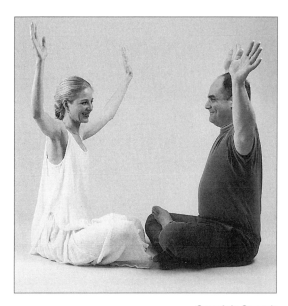

Couple's Stretch

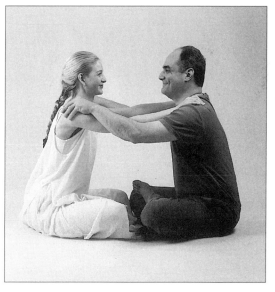

Couple's Massage

6. Facing your partner, stretch your arms in front of you, placing your hands on each other's shoulders. Massage each other and then relax.

Seeing Yourself in Your Partner

Start with preparatory steps one through four, as listed above. Then sit in Rock Pose (on your heels) facing your partner with your knees touching your partner's knees. Rest your hands in your lap in Venus Lock Mudra, in which the fingers are interlaced, palms facing each other. For men, the left little finger is on the bottom, and the right thumb is on top. For women, the left thumb is on top. For both, the inside thumb should press into the webbing between the forefinger and the thumb of the opposite hand. Fix your eyes on your partner's eyes. Concentrate on seeing your own image in your partner's eyes. Project love for 3 minutes. Then complete the kriya with steps one and two to end a Venus Kriya, as listed above.

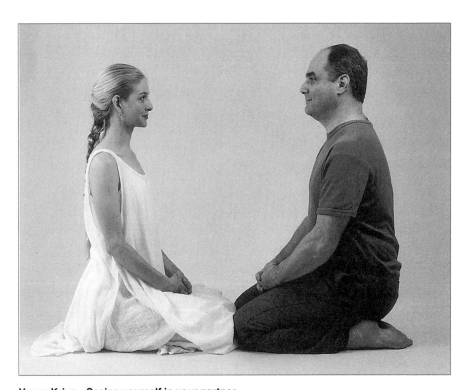

Venus Kriya—Seeing yourself in your partner

Benefits This is a powerful exercise that will help you become kind and compassionate toward your partner. It will help you to realize the true meaning of divine love.

Meditation to End an Argument

Do this meditation with your partner when you are arguing and cannot stop. It will break the spell of intolerance and confusion and help release anger. This kriya can help you maintain peace in your relationship and prevent situational anger from spreading to other areas of your lives.

Sit 4–5 feet from your partner in Easy Pose with a straight spine. Make fists of both hands. Put both fists with the back of your hands toward you, 6–8 inches in front of your third eye or brow point. Extend and press your thumb tips together until they become white (not too hard but with a firm pressure). Let the last joint of your thumb relax and bend as much as possible. Close your eyes.

With deep and powerful breaths, each partner alternates chanting the mantra while exhaling. Use the mantra of ecstasy, *Wha Hay Guroo* (pro-

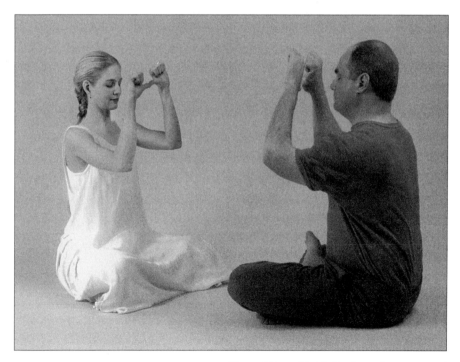

Venus Kriya—Meditation to end an argument

nounced *wha-hey goo-roo*), meaning "divine wisdom" or "ecstasy beyond time and space." Vibrate the pitch as high as you can. You should feel the vibration at your nose and brow point when you say *Guroo*. The sound *Wha Hay* lasts about 1 second, and the sound *Guroo* last about 7 seconds.

Listen to the sound of your partner chanting. If you concentrate and the sound is correct, you will feel it vibrate in you. Keep your eyes closed. Continue the chanting for 2 minutes. This meditation has the power to help you transcend your individual ego and attachments and to remember the union between you and your partner, and between you and the divine. When you finish the meditation, go to steps five and six as listed above, and relax.

Venus Life-Nerve Stretch

Sit opposite your partner on the floor, both of you stretching your legs out toward each other. Have your feet touching the feet of your partner, legs straight. Lean forward from your hips, keeping your spine lengthened as in a forward bend, and grasp the hands of your partner. Hold the posture with eyes open, looking into your partner's eyes as you project divine love to each other. Continue with relaxed breathing for 1 minute, then do Breath of Fire for 2 minutes. To end, inhale and suspend your breath (hold it in without straining). Exhale and apply the Root Lock. Follow with steps one and two as listed above for completing a Venus Kriya, then relax.

Foods for Sexuality

A wonderful home-cooked, fragrant meal can be a great beginning to a sexy evening. Fill the meal, and your home, with potent aromas—choose those that are subtle yet strong. Try cooking your favorite dishes with spices and herbs. Rest after the meal, then walk together and enjoy the foreplay, building toward your sexual union later in the night. The following foods have long been considered to support female sexuality. Enjoy!

Eggplant Pakoras

Eggplant is considered a very sensual food for women. According to the science of Ayurveda (Indian medical model), it is the most potent food for sup-

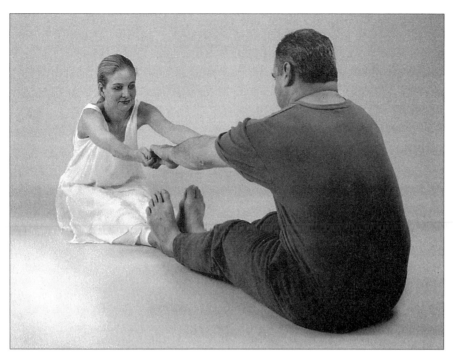

Venus Kriya—Life-Nerve Stretch

porting the female glandular system and regulating menstrual flow. To correct amenorrhea, or absence of your period, eat half an eggplant daily. This delicious Indian recipe includes garbanzo flour, which is also considered to be very healthy.

1 eggplant	1 tsp. black pepper
1 tbsp. caraway seeds	$^1/_2$ tsp. ground cloves
1 tsp. oregano seeds	$^3/_4$ cup onion juice or puree
1 tsp. cardamom pods	$^1/_2$ cup milk
2 cups garbanzo flour	$^1/_3$ cup water
$^1/_2$ tsp. cinnamon	$^1/_4$ cup honey
2 tsp. turmeric	Vegetable oil or ghee for frying
2 tsp. salt	

Cut the eggplant crosswise into about ⅜-inch-thick slices and set aside. Mix the seeds, pods, and spices with the garbanzo flour. Add onion juice, milk, water, and honey, and stir into paste; mix with fork until smooth. Dip the eggplant slices in the batter and fry in vegetable oil or ghee until golden brown. Transfer to paper towels to drain. Serve with catsup or chutney.

Serves 4–6.

Mangoes

Mango is a yogini food that enhances sex and that works as a medicine in every area of her life. If you have less milk when you are nursing, start eating mangoes, and your milk production will increase. If you have menstrual troubles, eat mangoes. For nausea in the early months of pregnancy, try a mango pickle. Take the skin off the pickle, put it on your upper palate, and just suck it with your tongue to keep yourself from vomiting or feeling nausea.

If you've never eaten a fresh mango, choose a ripe one that is somewhat soft, not too green, and has no obvious brown, bruised spots. Peel off the outside skin with a knife (it can be tough), then slice the fruit off the large oblong pit in the middle and cut it into pieces.

Yoga Practice with Your Partner to Enhance Your Senses and Sexuality

1. Tune in.

2. Long, Deep Breathing for 3 minutes.

3. Breath of Fire for 3 minutes.

4. Spinal Flex and Spinal Twist.

5. Venus Kriyas—choose one or two of the kriyas to practice with your partner.

6. Relax together to uplifting mantra music.

7. End with a prayer together.

Yoga Practice for Women

Full-body self-massage and cold shower hydrotherapy daily (except during menstruation and pregnancy). Add any scent to the high-quality oil you use. Try different scents and feel the effects of each (lavender for relaxation, citrus for stimulation, sandalwood for enhancing sexuality).

1. Tune in.

2. Choose any yoga set that addresses issues in your life (e.g., for balancing your cycle, increasing spinal flexibility, self-healing, or glandular health).

3. Practice the Body Locks. Inhale, exhale, and apply *Mula Bhanda,* the Root Lock. Repeat three times. Inhale, exhale, and apply *Mula Bhanda,* the Great Lock (combining the Root Lock, Diaphragm Lock, and Neck Lock). Practice this three times.

4. Practice Sat Kriya for balancing your chakras, balancing sexual energy, releasing stress, and clearing your mind. Or practice Kirtan

Kriya to help balance your Moon Centers and release fears and negative imprints of past sexual encounters.

5. Follow with deep relaxation to help you integrate the benefits of the yoga set.

6. To end, project a prayer for healing and love. Pray for yourself, the world, and anyone in your life who needs healing.

QUESTIONS FOR FURTHER GROWTH

- What are your present attitudes toward your sexuality? Take the time to journal your attitudes and evaluate how they impact your sexuality.

- Are you satisfied with the quality of your sexual relationship with your partner? If not, can you and your partner move toward an enlightened view of sex and increase physical and spiritual enjoyment?

- Are you holding back, faking enjoyment, or experiencing pain during intercourse? How is this affecting your relationship with yourself and your partner? Can you begin the journey of healing these issues?

- Are you willing to take a risk and try some of the yogini sexual secrets? Which ones?

7

Pregnancy, Childbirth, and Postpartum

The purest thing in the world is the heart of the mother. . . . It can move the universe. It can cause an effect beyond limitation.

—YOGI BHAJAN

Conception, pregnancy, and childbirth are physical manifestations of the *Adi Shakti,* each woman's primal creative power. The desire to give birth and love is deep, both a strong biological drive and spiritual force. The conscious decision to join energies and bring the infinity of another soul into this life unites a couple not only through their physical act, but also through the infinity of love itself, God's gift of the unborn soul who will soon experience this earth plane.

Together, through this elevated experience, a child is conceived and nurtured in the woman's womb and born into the world. So, too, a new family is born. Yogi Bhajan says of this experience that marriage is the highest yoga and children are your karmic teachers. Partnership with your mate is your greatest spiritual discipline, and your child is the teacher from whom you will learn the lessons you need to move forward on your spiritual path. This is the yogic approach to family.

Yoga for Receptivity and Conception

If you're planning to have a baby, meditate and evaluate your physical, mental, and spiritual health. You are preparing your body for the process of creating new life: You are your baby's first home. Your body, your consciousness, and your mental state are the first impressions this soul will experience. You can prepare yourself both physically and spiritually for conception.

Visit your doctor to evaluate your present state of health and follow any recommendations for staying healthy during pregnancy. Imagine yourself pregnant, and visualize your body. The thought vibrations you create as you think about your body affect your chemistry. Fall in love with that image, that lovely rounded figure that surrounds your baby with physical nurturing and love. Become the open receiver of the seed and this new soul.

You can also spiritually prepare yourself for conception by becoming open and receptive. Practicing meditation, prayer, and visualization can stimulate receptivity, a primary feminine quality. Meditation prepares you mentally and physically to receive universal energy. When you experience this universal energy and acknowledge it in your thoughts, your internal energy will rise to match the quality of infinity within you. Yoginis call this "bringing heaven down to earth." One way to initiate this process is to stimulate the navel point with breathing, chanting, or exercise. While you meditate, your thoughts will become calm, and you will link your finite self with infinity. Your meditative "call" invites the vibration of the infinite universe to meet you in your human form. Your energy rises, your chakras become stimulated, and you begin to feel energized and balanced. As soon as you decide to conceive, meditate daily and pull the heavens to you. This will create a receptivity that can assist your conception.

Prayer is different from meditation. Meditation opens you so that you can receive, whereas in prayer, you consciously ask the universe to listen and respond. Prayer energetically changes your entire being and can provide solace when you feel alone and exhausted. After each yoga practice session, or any time you feel the need, send your prayers out into the universe: Bless someone you love, heal yourself and others in your thoughts. Energy will follow your intention and awareness; your thoughts and projections will travel to their destination. Meditation and prayer can bring relaxation to the mind and body and increase the likelihood of conception.

Many women today struggle with the pain of *infertility*—the inability to become pregnant or maintain pregnancy. This pain is deeply felt and traumatic. There are many choices to be discussed with your doctor and partner, if you find yourself in this situation. Keep meditating and doing yoga, as it helps keep you connected during a time when you may feel isolated. If you decide on treatments involving hormone therapy, meditation can be an important component of your self-care program.

Conception

Previously, we presented the yogic view of sexuality as a sacred act. Sex can be especially meaningful if you are planning to conceive. You can also meditate before intercourse together. This can be particularly helpful if you are struggling with infertility and you begin to see sex as "something you have to do" and "something that isn't working." Try to enjoy your time together and let your body take the time to get stimulated so you can relax into intercourse.

Once you conceive, your life changes profoundly! Your thoughts turn toward caring for your baby and the security of your family. According to the philosophy of Kundalini Yoga, the soul of the child enters the body of the unborn fetus at 120 days. Prior to conception and the 120-day marker, it is advised that women meditate deeply and engage in excellent self-care. Both before and after 120 days, the physical, mental, and spiritual vibrations of the mother have a direct and lasting effect on her developing baby. The words you say, your thoughts, the foods you eat, and the situations you participate in influence your baby. Within the pregnant woman, the future generations of the world are being created. Even though pregnancy is an important foundation for your baby's future and should be taken seriously, it is meant to be enjoyed! Enjoy your life and try to relax and prepare for the changes in your body, mind, and lifestyle.

One-Minute Breath for Relaxing and Receptivity

Practice the One-Minute Breath before intercourse if you wish to become receptive and to conceive. Sit in Easy Pose (cross-legged) or in a comfortable position. Relax your hands into Gyan Mudra, with your thumbs touching your index fingers (making a circle) and your wrists resting on your knees.

Inhale slowly, taking 5 seconds to come to a full breath. Suspend (hold) your breath comfortably for 5 seconds. Exhale slowly, taking the full 5 seconds to complete the exhalation. Repeat the process. Keep your breath relaxed without straining on the inhalation, the breath suspension, or the exhalation. Do not hold the breath out. After you exhale, begin to inhale slowly again. Continue for 3–11 minutes. To end, inhale smoothly and deeply, briefly suspend your breath and focus on your brow point between your eyes and up, then exhale and relax.

Take your time building up this practice. If you become efficient, you may be able to move up to the maximum for this practice: inhaling for 20 seconds, suspending for 20 seconds, and exhaling for 20 seconds.

Benefits Whenever you are in a stressful state, your breath rate is quickened and your exhalation is incomplete. The One-Minute Breath helps slow your breath rate, which relieves the stress in your body and calms your mind. Of special note: Once you are pregnant, avoid holding or suspending your breath for long periods of time.

DR.'S NOTES *Stress, Science, and Pregnancy*

When a woman is pregnant, her metabolism and mental faculty go through tremendous changes. There is a life within the life, and it takes a lot of doing to keep the outer life, the woman, and the inner life, the child, in a balanced state.

—Yogi Bhajan

Is genetics or the environment the greater shaper of our destiny? Are we the sum of our genes or just some of our genes? With the mapping of the human genome, the cloning of animals, and the ability to identify major diseases by detecting a mistake in the structure or location of just one gene, most people are now aware of the powerful role that genetics plays in all of our lives. But what is the role of the environment? How powerful a role can it play when all the genes seem normal? How can yoga help?

There is no better model than pregnancy to answer these questions. Once a woman becomes pregnant, her life and the life of her developing baby are intricately interwoven. The mother's environment affects the child in both favorable and unfavorable ways. Many studies have linked stress during pregnancy with prematurity and low birth weight, both of which cause serious risk to the newborn. Pregnant women under significant psychological stress gain less weight than expected for the amount of calories they consume, probably as a result of the effects of stress on metabolism. This helps explain why pregnant women who experience severe stress during pregnancy deliver lower-birth-weight infants.

For example, pregnant women in especially stressful medical jobs produce higher levels of stress hormones than do women in less taxing jobs, although the study conducted was too small to show whether they also had a higher rate of complications. Similarly, pregnant enlisted women on active duty in the military are more likely to develop high blood pressure during pregnancy and to deliver low-birth-weight babies than nonworking wives of active-duty personnel.

Attitudes about work also matter. For instance, pregnant women who want to stop working are far more stressed than those who want to work, and such stress causes a significantly greater risk of preterm and low-birth-weight deliveries. Under whatever circumstances stress occurs, feeling trapped and helpless in a stressful situation is as important a determination for experiencing stress as the stress itself. According to Dr. Esther Sternberg in her book *The Balance Within* (New York: W. H. Freeman, 2000), less than 50 percent of our stress-responsiveness is in our genes, and more than 50 percent is molded by our environment. For this reason, every pregnant mother should realize that her baby's exposure to stress during pregnancy might lower the set point of the stress-responsiveness programmed by the baby's genes after delivery.

Because of these realities, yoga can play an important positive role on both the mother and her baby during pregnancy and beyond. It can decrease the body's oxygen needs; slow down breathing, heart rate, and blood pressure (among patients with elevated blood pressure); and lower levels of stress—all outcomes that benefit the developing baby. Repeating mantras can help lift the spirit and lower the negativism created by poor relationships, bad work situations, or similar stresses. The patterns of yogic breathing are also useful tools throughout labor and delivery, when Long, Deep Breathing and Breath of Fire can be useful tools during and between contractions. Finally, the sense of control and balance that comes with practicing yoga can sooth you during the helpless and off-balance moments when not only the center of the body's gravity but also the center of the mind's gravity are momentarily lost. Nothing can prevent stressful situations from occurring, but yoga can help counter the body's response to them.

BEFORE YOU EXERCISE

Before starting any exercise program, consult your doctor and review the beginning yoga instructions found in Chapters 1–3 in this book. If you are already athletic and have been exercising, don't expect to keep up with your present level of exercise. Stay with your routine unless you feel fatigued, stressed, or uncomfortable. If you begin feeling short of breath, stop exercising to ensure optimum oxygen supply to your baby. As your body changes, you will experience increased weight, a new center of gravity, and increased estrogen and progesterone levels. These changes may cause your joints, tendons, and ligaments to loosen and become sore. If this happens, you can adjust your routine to relieve the resulting tension. Consult the table on page 129 to measure your weight gain during pregnancy; consult with your doctor if you feel you are not gaining enough weight or are gaining too much.

 If you have not been exercising and feel out of shape, now is the time to begin special exercises for pregnant women. Join a prenatal exercise or yoga class where you know the exercises will be suited to your pregnancy and level of fitness. Take your time and do not exercise to the point of fatigue or feeling out of breath. Enjoy the breathing exercises and relaxation techniques and start walking!

PREGNANCY WEIGHT RECORD

Step 1: Record your prepregnancy weight and your recommended weight gain in the boxes.

Step 2: Place your current weight in the "Weight" column next to the appropriate "Week" of pregnancy (on the weeks when you do weigh-in).

Step 3: Calculate the total number of pounds you have gained (or lost) by subtracting your prepregnancy weight from your current weight. Record this number in the "Total" column. Repeat this calculation each time you weigh-in to keep a running total of your total pregnancy weight gain.

Prepregnancy Weight   Recommended Weight Gain

First Trimester			Second Trimester			Third Trimester		
Week	Weight	Total	Week	Weight	Total	Week	Weight	Total
1			13			26		
2			14			27		
3			15			28		
4			16			29		
5			17			30		
6			18			31		
7			19			32		
8			20			33		
9			21			34		
10			22			35		
11			23			36		
12			24			37		
			25			38		
						39		
						40		

Walking

According to Kundalini Yoga (and many medical professionals), the best exercise for a woman during pregnancy is walking 2–5 miles every day. Start with a 20-minute walk and try to increase your time by 5 minutes daily until you reach at least 1 hour. While you walk, make sure most of the impact occurs on the balls of your feet. In yoga it is called walking on your "paws." (This way of walking can be used in power walking as well.) When your heel hits the ground, keep your foot pointing straight ahead. Roll over your heel, following the outside edge of your foot, onto the balls of your feet. Push your weight onto the balls of your foot to propel you into the next step. Walking like this can relieve back and knee stress and give you more energy!

You may get tired during your walk, especially if the incline is steep. For that reason, it is best to walk on a flat surface or on no more than a one-degree incline if you walk on a treadmill. Take a break, stretch, and enjoy the fresh air until you are rested. Use an inside track, a treadmill, or a large shopping mall if the weather is inclement or it is icy. Walk with other pregnant women to stay motivated, supported, and socially involved, and to have fun!

You can add a meditative quality to walking by listening to uplifting tapes or mentally chanting. Try walking with your spouse and chanting the mantra *Sat Naam* as the left foot hits the ground, and *Wha Hay Guroo* as your right foot hits the ground. Chanting aloud affects your glandular system in a positive way and relaxes your mind.

Swimming

From the yogic perspective, water is a primary healer for women. Playing and splashing in the water help release tension and calm your mood. It also feels great to be in the water, because all your weight is supported, which allows you to feel balanced as you exercise. The low-impact effects of swimming help keep the muscles in shape without putting stress on your joints, especially your back and knees. Walking backward and forward in the water can be great exercise. Or try slowly cycling your legs as you float: Stand with your back against the side of the pool, stretch your arms backward, and hold on to the side of the pool. An appropriate water aerobics class in your area might also be fun.

Posture

As you progress in your pregnancy, you may find it difficult to maintain your balance. The additional weight of the baby changes your center of gravity, which has an impact on your posture. To help you adjust for this, correct your posture as often as possible. Good posture and support will help you to

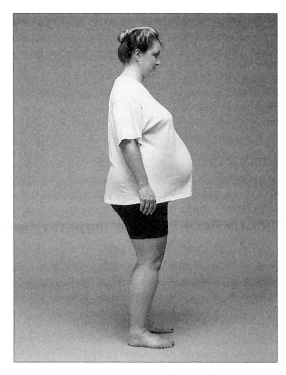

Posture for pregnancy

feel better and to move more easily throughout your pregnancy. (See the illustration above for an example of proper posture.) Instead of leaning back and arching your spine, lengthen and straighten your back. Instead of leaning left or right, center the baby and support your weight with your thighs and buttocks, keeping your knees bent slightly. Lift your chest at the sternum (breast bone) and let your shoulders relax. Stand with your feet apart so you feel steady and supported. Practice this each morning and throughout the day to prevent back stiffness and to maximize energy. Some women find that using a corset specially designed to support a pregnant uterus helps them maintain good posture without strain.

Relaxing Breathing Techniques for Pregnancy

Your yoga practice is a time to appreciate the universal process of creativity and to consciously relax. When you are relaxed, your baby will sense your love and enter a relaxed state as well. It's best to practice in a cozy place with plenty of fresh air. Having a mat and cushion to sit on will help support your lower back. (Be sure to refrain from any posture or exercise that is uncomfortable for you.) You are free to use any of the meditation and relaxation techniques in this book that appeal to you during pregnancy. However, do not choose any that strain your breathing, include Breath of Fire, or use the abdominal muscles for pumping the belly. Otherwise, enjoy discovering the ones that work for you.

When you begin, tune in (see "Yoga Basics" in Chapter 2) and take a few breaths to bring your focus to your body. Mentally repeat the mantra *Sat Naam* on each breath to focus your mind throughout your practice, staying especially sensitive to any messages your body gives you.

Deep Breathing

As your baby grows, your diaphragm muscle will have less space to flex as you breathe, which may make it harder to see your belly rise and fall with each breath. Avoid transitioning to a shallow breathing pattern. When you do Long, Deep Breathing, the rib cage doesn't *lift;* rather it *expands* to the sides. You are still using your diaphragm to breath but feeling most of the sensation from your midsection up to your ribs. When you breathe correctly, your shoulders, neck, and chest muscles will feel relaxed rather than strained.

To practice deep breathing, put the back of your hands underneath your armpits and against your rib cage. Inhale and feel the rib cage press against your hands. As you exhale, feel the rib cage return and relax. Feel the rhythm of the breath and use the mantra *Sat* on the inhalation and *Naam* on the exhalation. Teach your mind to focus and relax by allowing the mantra to cut through any negative or distracting thoughts. Your body and baby will benefit from increased circulation, increased oxygenation, and released stress and anxiety. Try 11 minutes of this technique any time you feel restless, anxious, or overwhelmed. If you feel tired and need to nap, Long, Deep Breathing will bring you to a restful sleep.

Segmented Breathing

Sitting in Easy Pose (cross-legged), take a few Long, Deep Breaths. Then begin inhaling in four short segments and exhaling in four segments. As a variation, inhale four segments and exhale in one long unbroken breath. Breathe through the nose and go at a pace that is comfortable; you should not feel strained or out of breath. Continue for 1–3 minutes, or up to 11 minutes, and then relax. You can try other breath ratios, such as inhaling eight segments, then exhaling eight segments, etc. Link your breath with the mantra *Saa Taa Naa Maa.*

Benefits Segmented breathing works quickly to relax you by slowing your breath rate and to energize you by intensifying your focus and awareness. This type of breathing also safely exercises your abdominal muscles. They move slightly with each segment, stretching with the inhalation and moving toward your spine with the exhalation. Many women find that segmented breathing revitalizes their energy and relieves stressful thoughts.

Yoga Exercises for Pregnancy

Butterfly Stretch

Sit on a level surface and bring the soles of your feet together in front of your groin. Hold your feet with your hands, fingers interlaced. Let the knees relax and straighten your spine. Relax your neck and keep your chin tucked toward your neck. Breathe slow Long, Deep Breaths, feeling your rib cage open to the sides as you inhale, and feeling it relax as you exhale. While you breathe, slowly bounce the knees up and down, creating a fluttering motion. These movements are small. Bring your attention to your groin and the stretch you feel in your thighs and hips. Keep your breath relaxed throughout. Continue the motion for 1–3 minutes.

Benefits This exercise relaxes and stretches the hips, legs, and thighs, and strengthens the pelvic floor. The Butterfly Stretch helps to prepare the pelvic floor for birth by bringing greater flexibility and circulation to the area. Keeping your back straight during the exercise will help strengthen back muscles to support the extra weight of the baby. Do this stretch anytime you feel nervous or tight, and it will help you to relax.

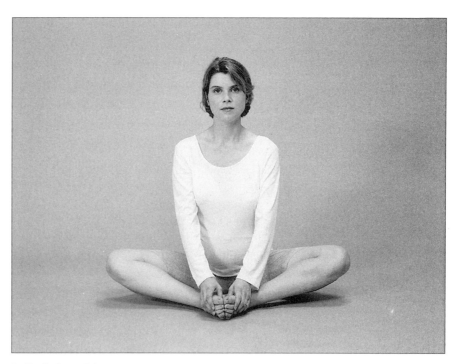

Butterfly Stretch for pregnancy

Pregnancy Life-Nerve Stretch

Sit on the floor with your legs stretched out in front of you. Spread your legs apart (about 2–3 feet or as far apart as you can, still sitting upright). Sit with your spine erect and stretch your arms out in front of you, parallel to the floor. Inhale and lean slightly back. Exhale and lean forward, stretching your arms and keeping them parallel to the floor. Create a rhythmic movement, mentally chanting *Sat* when you inhale and *Naam* when you exhale. Continue for up to 3 minutes.

Benefits This exercise stretches the backs of your legs, your groin, and your lower back, increasing circulation and flexibility. It also helps keep your back strong throughout your pregnancy, relieves constipation and gas, and relaxes your nerves. In yoga, we call the sciatic nerve along the back of the legs the "life nerve" because of the effect stretching this area has on the entire nervous system. When you keep this area flexible, you release tension in all areas of

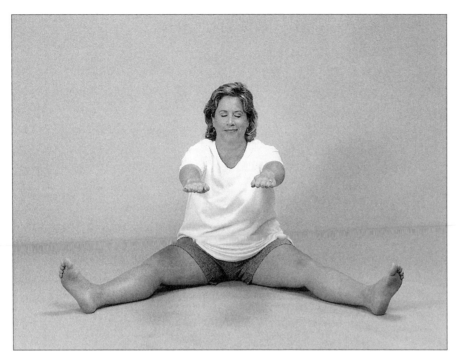

Pregnancy Life-Nerve Stretch

your body and mind, which relaxes you deeply and can improve your sleep. One cautionary note: If you are already experiencing *sciatica*—inflammation of the sciatic nerve—do **not** do this stretching exercise until the pain is totally gone.

Basic Spinal Flex

Begin by sitting cross-legged on the floor or in a chair. Hold on to your shins with your hands. As you inhale, sit straight or flex your spine forward slightly, mentally chanting *Sat.* As you exhale, relax your spine back, holding on to your shins for steadiness and mentally chant *Naam.* Continue in a rhythmic motion, inhaling forward and exhaling as you go back. Move continuously and smoothly at a steady speed without stopping. Use a distinct breath, filling your lungs about one-quarter of the way on the inhalation, and exhaling an equal amount. Use the mantra to focus your mind.

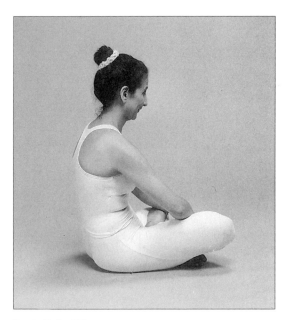

Basic Spinal Flex

Benefits The spinal flex is wonderful for stretching your lower and upper back. The exercise creates a comforting rhythm that increases flexibility and releases tension and pain.

Squatting—To Prepare for Birthing

Squatting is a helpful exercise for pregnancy. You can begin with your back against a wall or with a sturdy chair in front of you for support. Squat down and maintain the position for as long as is comfortable. (Start with 1 minute a few times a day and build *slowly*.) Breathe Long, Deep Breaths, relaxing your body. Hold the chair for support. If you need to, place a folded towel or blanket under your heels for support. To come out of the squat, stand slowly, so you do not get dizzy. You can also end the squat by sitting fully on the floor. You can then relax or stand up without pressure on your knees.

Benefits Women around the world often find squatting the most comfortable posture for giving birth as well as for socializing and waiting for the bus! It is said that the women of many cultures who practice this posture their whole lives have a much easier time giving birth, as this exercise increases flexibility and circulation of the pelvic area, and strengthens and stretches your back and legs. You can squat to get down to floor level to pick something up, play with children, or when you need to bend over or lift something. Squatting also helps elimination and can help prevent constipation and hemorrhoids. *Caution:* Do **not** practice squatting if your doctor has indicated to you that your cervix is soft or opened before term.

Pelvic Floor Exercises (Kegels)

Pelvic floor exercises can be done at any time. To practice, sit comfortably and relax your breath. Tighten your bladder muscles (as if you are stopping the flow of your urine). Hold for a moment, then let go gradually. Think of

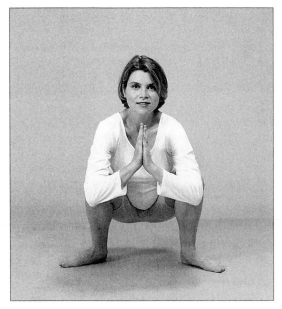

Squatting to prepare for birthing, early in pregnancy

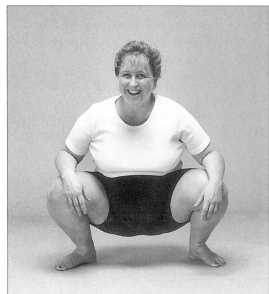

Squatting to prepare for birthing, later in pregnancy

this movement like that of an elevator, drawing the muscle up to the top floors, holding for a maximum of 10 seconds, then slowly releasing, letting the elevator back down to the ground floor. Do these exercises as often as you wish. Practice after you have emptied your bladder.

Benefits This exercise can quickly help you strengthen the muscles of the pelvic floor, preventing loss of urine during coughing or sneezing. Don't underestimate this common and simple exercise. Many women report increased strength after only a few weeks of practicing it about fifty times a day.

Exercises for Upper Body and Breasts

These exercises help maintain strong circulation in the breast area. They also help relax any tension that accumulates from stress or swollen and increased breast size. Keeping the muscles in the breast area strong is a benefit throughout pregnancy and nursing.

Shoulder Lifts and Circles

Start by sitting in Easy Pose (cross-legged) on the floor or in a chair. Inhale and bring your shoulders up, then exhale, relaxing the shoulders down again. Do not strain or stretch to the point of stress. Do the exercise rhythmically with your breath. It is a relatively quick movement with a segmented breath (about 80–100 shrugs per minute). The object of this exercise is to bring circulation and movement to your shoulders, *not* necessarily to really stretch them. Think of it as *shoulder dancing*! Keep your chin relaxed and parallel to the floor so your neck will be relaxed. Continue for 1–3 minutes. To end the exercise, inhale and hold the shoulders in a shrugged position briefly, then exhale as you relax.

Still sitting in Easy Pose, begin rolling your shoulders forward while breathing in Long, Deep Breaths. Roll forward for 1–3 minutes, then roll backward for 1–3 minutes. Make sure your neck stays relaxed by keeping your chin tucked toward your neck and parallel to the floor.

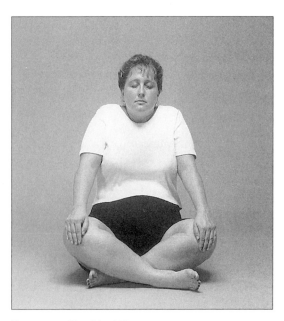

Pregnancy Shoulder Lifts

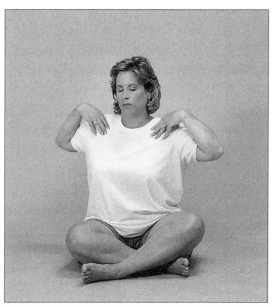

Pregnancy Spinal Twist

Upper Spinal Twist—For Back and Breasts

Start this exercise in Easy Pose or sitting in a chair. Place your hands on your shoulders, fingers in front and thumbs in back. Twist left while inhaling and right while exhaling, moving your torso and head together. Inhale and exhale in short segments, maintaining a smooth rhythm. Keep your elbows out and up, even with your shoulders and parallel to the floor. Do not stretch to your maximum, and if you feel dizzy, go slower. Feel the rhythm of the breath and body and keep the motion smooth and continuous, about fifteen twists every 30 seconds. Continue for up to 3 minutes maximum.

Benefits These exercises help improve circulation in the breast area, keep your shoulders flexible and relaxed, and release any tension that accumulates from swollen, enlarged breasts. The spinal twisting exercise can also help strengthen the upper back, to give your muscles additional circulation, and help prevent headaches.

Exercise Set for Pregnancy

This exercise set incorporates many excellent postures that all work together for pregnancy. Do these exercises together as a set or as individual practices.

1. ***Breathe—Arms Out.*** Sit in a comfortable posture on the floor or in a chair. Lengthen your spine and sit straight without strain. Hold your arms out to your sides, parallel to the floor. Hold this posture for 3–5 minutes with slow Long, Deep Breathing. Relax.

2. ***Spinal Flex.*** Do this exercise as described previously in this chapter for 1–3 minutes. To end, inhale, straighten your spine, then exhale and relax.

3. ***Butterfly Stretch.*** Do this exercise for 1 minute as described previously in this chapter. Then massage your inner thighs with your hands for 1 minute. Bring the soles of your feet together again and bounce your knees gently for 1 more minute.

4. ***Hip Stretch.*** Stretch your legs straight out, and spread them apart from each other as wide as is comfortable. You should still be able to sit up

comfortably. Lean forward and grasp your toes, or let your hands rest on your shins or knees. Inhale and gently stretch your spine up, still holding your toes, or resting your hands on your legs. Exhale and stretch gently forward, feeling the stretch in your hips. Repeat a few times.

5. *Pelvic Tilt.* Crouch on the floor on your hands and knees. As you inhale, lift your head and look straight ahead while keeping your back parallel to the floor. As you exhale, relax your head down, pulling in your stomach muscles and tightening your buttocks, and tilt your pelvis forward and under. Your back will arch up, the area between the shoulder blades stretching toward the ceiling. Do not bend your elbows as you do the exercise. If your wrists are stiff, make a fist and hold your wrists straight with weight on your fist. Continue the movement slowly and rhythmically with breath and mantra for 1–3 minutes, then relax.

Benefits The Pelvic Tilt can help release sciatic and lower-back tension and give your organs and bones a rest from carrying weight in an upright position. This exercise can be done in many positions, including lying down and standing up (see variations above). A nice addition is having your partner massage your lower back as you move slowly! Do this daily to remain flexible and relieve stress, and whenever you want relief from stiffness.

6. *Hip Rotation.* Crouching on your hands and knees, begin to rotate your hips in circles. Continue rotating your hips in one direction for 1–3 minutes. Pause and reverse the direction and continue for another 1–3 minutes.

7. *Relax into Baby Pose.* From the position of sitting on your heels, spread your knees, leaving room for your belly. Lean forward and rest your head on the floor. Relax your arms by your side, near your feet, with your palms facing upward. (This is Baby Pose.) Relax your breath and meditate at your brow point, just between your eyes. If you are experiencing low or high blood pressure or you get dizzy, place a mat under your head so that it does not go lower than your heart, or rest your head in your hands. Rest in this position for 3–5 minutes. Come out of the posture slowly and relax for a few moments before going to the next exercise.

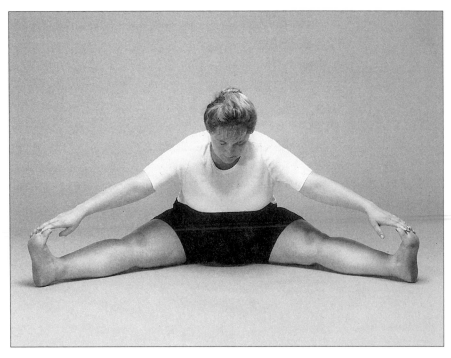

Pregnancy Hip Stretch

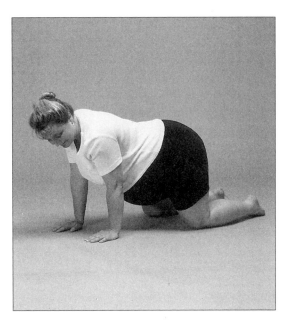

Pregnancy Cow

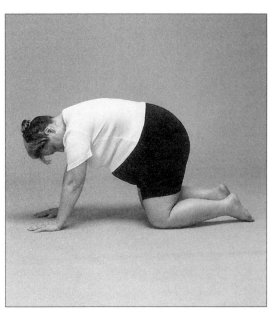

Pregnancy Cat

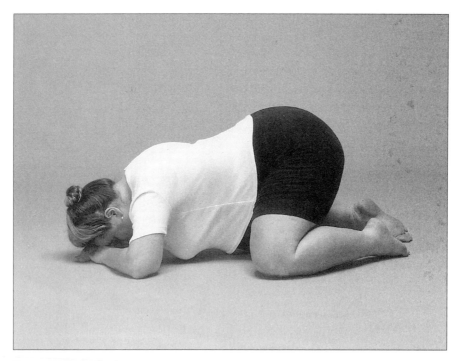

Pregnancy Baby Pose

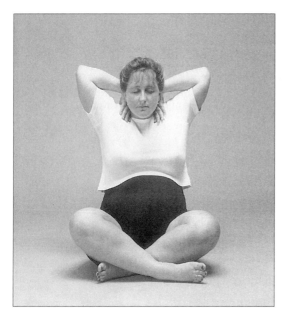

Pregnancy Elbow Lifts

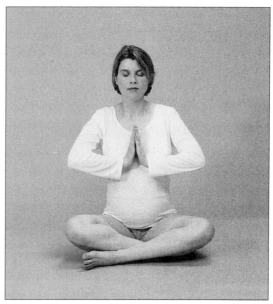

Pregnancy, palms pressed together

8. *Upper Spinal Twist.* Do this exercise as described previously in the chapter for 1–3 minutes. To end, inhale facing forward, and then relax.

9. *Elbow Lifts.* Bring your hands to your shoulders again, as in the previous posture. Inhale and lift your elbows up toward the sky, then exhale, bringing them down to your side. Continue this motion for 1–3 minutes. To end, inhale, stretch up, and hold briefly, then exhale and relax.

10. *Palms Pressed Together.* In a seated posture, press your palms together in front of your chest. Press firmly, holding the pressure without tensing your shoulders or neck. Continue holding this posture with Long, Deep Breathing for 1–3 minutes. Inhale and hold briefly, then exhale and relax.

11. *Pelvic Floor (Kegel) Exercise.* Sit in Easy Pose with your hands in Gyan Mudra (index fingers and thumbs together, making a circle) resting on your knees. Practice your pelvic floor exercises (Kegels), as previously described, for 3 minutes.

12. *Relax Deeply.* Relax in a position that is comfortable and supportive, such as on your side, with a pillow to support your head and legs.

Benefits This kriya is an excellent all-around workout for the pregnant women. It targets every potential problem area and will change your mood dramatically! Make sure to relax deeply after this set!

Relaxing, Meditating, and Talking to Your Baby

Staying relaxed is vital for remaining healthy and stable during the transitions of pregnancy, birth, and afterward. To maintain your stability, practice one meditation and one 11-minute relaxation each day, either on your own or after yoga class. After exercise, yoga, and each meditation, relax: Give your body the opportunity to integrate the positive changes you have worked for.

You can relax each part of your body by doing a systemic tensing and release of your muscles, starting from the feet and moving throughout the body until you feel all your muscles relax. Find a comfortable position for rest and become still. While you tense and relax, use your mind to send the message to all your muscles and inner organs that they can relax. Go to your highest consciousness and instruct your cells and entire body to become still. Inhale *Sat* and exhale *Naam,* allowing the repetition of the mantra to cut through any physical or mental tension.

Listen to some of the recommended relaxation tapes and find the technique that works for you. Use it daily. Learn to relax on command, a skill that will help you during labor and birthing. Using alternative nostril breathing (as described in Chapter 2) or the following breathing technique and meditation will help you develop the skill of relaxation.

Chanting Meditation—To Relax You and Your Baby

This meditation is a beautiful way to relax; it's like having a spiritual conversation with your baby. Sit in a comfortable meditation posture. Hold your hands so that the thumb of the left hand rests in the palm of the right. Cross the thumb of your right hand over the left thumb. Relax your elbows by your side and raise both hands so they are in front of your chest area. Eyes are closed. Inhale a Long, Deep Breath. On the exhalation, chant a long *Saaaaaat* (pronounced *su-u-u-ht,* as in the word *but*). At the very end, when your breath is almost all out, chant a short *Naam* just to let out the last parts of your breath. Pronounce *Sat* thirty-five times longer than *Naam* (in a ratio of 35:1). Inhale deeply and repeat the chant, allowing the voice to open and the breath to release slowly. Experience the sound. Do not struggle; let the sound be like a "call." Continue for 3–31 minutes. To end, inhale, suspend the breath briefly, then exhale and relax. In a short time you can be breathing 4–6 breaths per minute, down from the normal 12–15 breaths per minute.

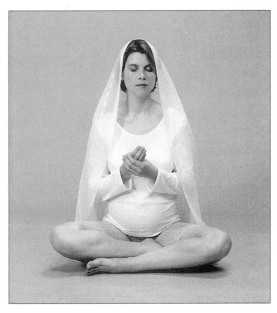

Pregnancy chanting meditation to relax you and your baby

Benefits The long exhalation as you chant the mantra enables your breathing to slow down. Your body and mind receive a message of calm from your slowing breath rate, allowing you and your baby to relax. *You both will fall in love with your voice and the sound of your call.* Try this meditation any time to help you find your balance and neutralize tension.

Healing Yourself and Your Baby

Pregnancy can be a healing experience for women. The essentially feminine sensations of pregnancy can be spiritually healing. Some women feel the passing of love from generation to generation. Others may feel old traumas resurface, and hope and pray they can break negative patterns of past generations and create a new reality of love. Meditation can help process your subconscious and release negative patterns as you create positive intentions and project a positive future for youself and your family.

You can begin to heal yourself and your baby by practicing any of the meditation techniques and relaxation exercises and by having conversations with the developing child within you. One technique for healing is the practice of *Sat Naam Rasayan.* This beautiful healing art can strengthen the loving relationship between you and your child within you and can deepen your experience of pregnancy by helping you stay in the present moment.

Sat Naam Rasayam

Sit in Easy Pose or in a comfortable position. Relax your breath.

1. ***Bring your attention to your bodily sensations.*** Notice all the parts of your body and how they are feeling. Some parts may be stiff, others relaxed. Some parts may be calling your attention to them, others draw hardly any notice. Include the sensation of your growing baby in your awareness, along with all the other sensations and feelings. Continue to sit and simply notice your sensations without placing too much attention on any one of them.

2. ***Include any thoughts you have in your sensations.*** Be aware of your thinking without letting any one thought distract you. Allow your thinking to flow without following any one thought. Many

thoughts come as you sit quietly, just as in meditation. Don't ignore them and don't let them pull you away from experiencing all your body sensations.

3. ***Maintain this mental state, becoming aware of all your sensations*** without allowing any one to monopolize your attention. Continue for a few minutes until you feel you are actually aware of all your sensations.

4. ***Feel all of your sensations simultaneously.*** This state is called *equalization*. As you experience your arm, you experience your back; as you experience your breath, you experience a thought. As you experience a thought, you experience your baby. The stage of equalization is a stage of expansion beyond the pull of body and mind. This expansion brings you beyond the duality of thinking and feeling into the heart of love and truth. Hold this attitude for a few minutes.

5. ***Project an intention while in this stage of equalization.*** Project the intention to release the stress you and your baby may be holding. Let the intention go as soon as you think it, then go back to equalizing your sensations. Sit for another few minutes. Then take a deep breath, stretch, and relax.

This healing technique helps you deepen your relationship with your baby, steady your nerves, and heal old wounds. Through practicing Sat Naam Rasayam, your heightened senses and intuition will lead you to emphasize the positive aspects of pregnancy and experience its deeper meaning.

Yoga and the Power of Your Mind—Giving Birth

Giving birth is the ultimate creative experience; no one can accurately predict the totality of the experience of your child's birth. Your attitude about giving birth will have a powerful impact on your experience.

It is natural to be fearful of any experience that is unknown and unpredictable, especially one as intense as childbirth. As you notice fears come up, go into your highest healing consciousness. Remember your yoga meditations. Use a positive healing thought, a picture, a mantra, or your child's name to help you return to the present moment. Work with your baby in the delivery process by breathing between contractions and surrendering to the experience of birth. Many yoga students find it helpful to practice visualizing their baby moving through the birth canal during birth. Other students report that their practice of relaxation and repeating mantras helps them focus their minds. Addressing fear, surrendering to the moment, and working with your baby and your body during the birthing process can help ensure that you will have a satisfying birth experience.

The Power of Breathing During Labor

Breathing for childbirth will help direct your attention and focus, keep you present in the moment, and help ease the stress you and your baby may feel. Managing labor is really about managing your breathing and your consciousness throughout the delivery experience. Long, Deep Breathing between contractions stimulates the pituitary gland and helps the secretion of oxytocin, which supports the contractions and the flow of oxygen to you and your baby.

Keep yourself hydrated during labor. It is advisable not to take any solid foods during active labor. Drink healthy beverages like pure water and gentle teas with honey in small sips. This can help you maintain your energy and comfort you. Keep the liquids you drink at room temperature or warmer to reduce any stress on your digestive system.

Use the power of your mind to create positive images of giving birth. Even though you may be feeling *contractions*, your body is also *expanding* and opening to deliver life into the world. Many cultures compare the birthing process to the blooming of a flower. You can place blooming flowers by your side as you give birth to remind you of this image.

Labor is stressful, but your body is taking control, so let it! Nature is in action. Continue to practice your relaxation techniques and breathing, even if you are experiencing difficulties and the birth is not going the way you anticipated. Keep your thoughts as spiritual and positive as possible. Especially with emergency procedures, staying in the present moment will assist your baby. By using visualization, practicing Long, Deep Breathing between contractions, and maintaining a positive mental attitude, you can channel the stress created by labor into the powerful energy of giving birth.

Postpartum

After the delivery you can hold your baby and spend this precious time together. If possible, have your partner nearby. Your baby will feel most secure if allowed to rest, relate to you, and nurse whenever needed. Most new mothers leave the hospital within 48 hours. If you are too tired or feeling uncertain, make sure you have the option of staying in the hospital if you need to. It is helpful for new mothers and fathers to have enough support once they get home to nurture the new family. Plan ahead.

Almost all new mothers experience sleep deprivation, especially if they are breast-feeding, because a new baby will be hungry almost every 3 hours. Medically, breast-feeding is healthy for new mothers and new babies. Not only does it create a special feeling of closeness, but suckling also stimulates the glandular system to help shrink the uterus to its normal size, and breast milk contains antibodies that help protect your baby from certain illnesses.

There is also a value in community. If you don't have or can't afford child care, seek out friends and family to help you, even for short windows of time.

The yogis believe that the mother and baby still share one aura at the time of birth and for 40 days after birth. The first 40 days of a baby's life is a time for the immediate family to bond and create a secure environment for the baby. The importance of these first 40 days cannot be overstated. Both you and your baby need attention, rest, and security during this time. Your baby is acclimating to the world, and you are recovering from the birthing experience. Rest, meditate, and bond with your baby.

As a new mother you may experience a range of emotions. You may feel elated and ecstatic at times, and sad at other times. Sleep deprivation and a lack of support may also cause you to feel depressed or overwhelmed. According to Dr. Arlene Huysman in her book *A Mother's Tears,* 80 percent of women who give birth experience some form of postpartum upset, and 20–40 percent of these report significant emotional disturbance. A much smaller percentage report severe or debilitating symptoms known as postpartum depression. Don't suffer silently if you become fatigued or fearful. The first 6 weeks postpartum is considered a time of recovery for your body. It is too early to resume strenuous exercise, but it is an excellent time to return to practicing meditation and relaxation.

Mother Is the First Teacher

Once you have given birth, you become your child's first teacher. Your child looks to you for guidance, honesty, and unconditional love. Don't underestimate the sensitivity of a new baby. The child not only hears your voice and understands your vibration, but also senses the subtlest energies around him or her. Being a yogini mother means understanding this sensitivity and committing to nurturing the child into a self-sufficient being with the values and strength to face the challenges of life. This is the time to keep up your yoga practice. Don't give up because you are busy; keep your baby with you as you practice. Meditate and chant while breast-feeding. Meditate while your baby is napping, if only for 5 minutes. Every morning, arise with gratitude, even if you are tired. After you arise, take a cold shower if possible, and then adopt a positive attitude to meet your baby with a smile. Every smile gives your baby self-assurance and the experience of your love.

Postpartum Yoga and Exercise

Do not start a full Kundalini Yoga exercise routine until 3 months after giving birth. Begin exercising slowly with Pelvic Floor (Kegel) exercises and Long, Deep Breathing. After a few weeks, start walking to massage your organs. Exercise outdoors if possible. Listen to your body; do not overwork too soon. After 2 weeks, you can try these exercises:

1. Lie on your back. Cross your legs at your ankles, squeeze your pelvic floor and buttock muscles, and squeeze your thighs together. Raise your head and count to five, then relax. Repeat the exercise ten times, twice daily. This will help strengthen your abdomen.

2. Lie on your back with your legs stretched out. Lift one knee slightly, leaving your foot still on the floor. With your opposite arm, try to stretch and reach your bent knee. Hold the position for a count of five. Relax and then repeat with the other side. It's okay if you do not reach your knee; it's the stretch that is important. You are stretching the diagonal abdominal muscles. You can do this exercise ten times on each side twice a day.

3. Lie on your back. Bend your knees to your chest. Rest your hands under your back at the base of your spine. Squeeze your buttock muscles and press your abdominal muscles down toward the floor. Rock your pelvis so your back goes flat to the floor. Lift your head up and to your chest until your abdominal muscles tighten and contract. Repeat this exercise ten times twice a day.

Postpartum Suggestions

Massage your uterus every half-hour after birth and every 2–3 hours during the first 24 hours after giving birth. Use the heel of your hand, massaging in a downward direction.

Be positive, meditate gently, and relax. Think positive thoughts and use mantras, chants, and uplifting songs to nurture the spirit of both you and your baby. Take a nap after you finish breast-feeding. Relaxation can help you to produce better milk.

Yogis recommend at least two 1-hour naps each day during the first 40 days after giving birth. Allow yourself and your family the privacy to relax and adjust during this time.

Special Recipes for New Mothers

Milk Production Tea

Boil equal amounts of fennel seeds, anise seeds, and cumin seeds for 10 minutes. Strain before drinking.

Special Nursing Mother's Drink

6 oz. milk

6–8 blanched almonds, soaked and peeled

2 tbsp. ghee (clarified butter)

1–2 tsp. honey

Blend well and drink once a day.

Tapioca

$1/2$ cup tapioca (large pearls)

2 cups milk

$1/4$ cup or less honey

YOGIC DIET FOR NEW MOTHERS

- Drink plenty of water.

- Ginger tea is a tonic that strengthens nerves and is said to help milk production. Add milk and honey to taste.

- Drink two glasses or more of milk daily, if you are breast-feeding.

- Try these healing foods for after childbirth: sautéed almonds, mung beans and rice (well cooked), tapioca (high in protein, easy to digest, and prevents constipation, but do not use instant).

- Eat a balanced diet that includes lots of fresh foods.

- Eat fresh fruits for vitamin C. Fresh carrot juice can be healthy postpartum if you do not find it too sweet for you.

- Avoid hot spices, raw onions and garlic, cabbage (even broccoli), and dried or fresh beans that can produce gas. Avoid chocolate, as it can produce gas in newborns through your milk. Use healthy dressings that include cold-pressed oils to make raw vegetables more digestible.

- To help constipation, try to walk and eat well to get your digestive system moving. Take an enema if you need to.

- Keep a Thermos of Yogi Tea by your bed. Drink Yogi Tea often to boost your energy and overall vitality.

Soak tapioca pearls in water for 6–12 hours before cooking (soak smaller pearls for less time, and larger pearls for longer time). Combine all ingredients in a saucepan and cook over medium heat until mixture thickens and tapioca becomes clear. Add the honey at the beginning or the pudding may become too thin.

Mung Beans and Rice See recipe in Chapter 9. Note: Lessen or eliminate spices so that the mung beans are mild.

Yoga for Receptivity

1. Tune in.

2. Long, Deep Breathing for 3 minutes in Easy Pose (cross-legged).

3. Spinal Flex and Spinal Twist, twenty-six times.

4. Pregnancy Life-Nerve Stretch for 1–3 minutes.

5. One-Minute Breath: inhale 5 seconds, suspend 5 seconds, and exhale 5 seconds continuously for 3–62 minutes.

6. Relax on your back for 11 minutes, arms by your sides and palms facing upward.

7. Grace of God Meditation.

QUESTIONS FOR FURTHER GROWTH

- Are you receptive in your life? You can compare this with being controlling, defensive, or fearful. Are you open to receive what life brings?

- Are you prepared to attract a new soul into your life?

- Can you schedule two sessions of relaxation each day, of 11 minutes each, if you are pregnant? If not, how do you relax and take time to nurture yourself and your baby?

- Physically giving birth is one manifestation of your creativity and femininity. What are the other areas in your life in which you "give birth" and manifest your creativity?

Yoga for Pregnancy

Any time you feel the need to calm down, center, or focus, choose to project a positive thought or take a moment to do the healing exercise. Look for times to integrate yoga into your day, such as when you are waiting in the doctor's office or when you have a few minutes during a break at work. Create the habit of being in a positive relationship with your baby.

1. Tune in.

2. Long, Deep Breathing and/or segmented breathing for 1–3 minutes.

3. Spinal Flex, with soles of your feet together and holding your ankles, twenty-six times.

4. Spinal Twist, twenty-six times.

5. Butterfly.

6. Life-Nerve Stretch.

7. Squat.

8. Mantra Meditation for 3–11 minutes to Relax You and Your Baby.

9. Relax.

10. Healing Exercise.

11. Projection and conversation with your baby.

If you have more time, you can do the entire set of yoga exercises as listed in Chapter 7.

Yoga and Walking for Pregnancy

1. Tune in.

2. Spinal Flex and Spinal Twist.

3. Walking for 15 minutes to a maximum of 5 miles. Try the *Charn Jaap,* mentally chanting as you walk with your partner or friend.

4. When your walk is complete, either relax, meditate, or do the Healing Exercise.

5. Project a positive affirmation or a prayer, and initiate a conversation with your baby.

- What are your prayers and hopes for your child?

- While pregnant, you are the mother, but once your child is born, some describe your role as that of the teacher. How are you a mother to the baby inside your womb? When your child is born, how will you be the teacher? What is the difference between these roles?

- Do you relax twice a day, for 11 minutes each, and talk to your baby? If not, how can you arrange your schedule to include these practices?

Yoga for Postpartum

1. Tune in.

2. Grace of God Meditation.

3. Chanting with your baby.

4. Healing Exercise, chanting (aloud or silently), and projecting positive intentions and prayers while holding or breast-feeding your baby.

5. Relax.

Yoga is the state of being present in your experience. Until you can begin an exercise program, use the techniques you have learned to continue to relax both you and your baby. Don't give up; you can do these exercises for even a few minutes in bed, if needed. Your relaxed mental state will create a loving home and positively affect your loved ones.

If your baby is crying or fidgety for no obvious reason, and you are exhausted, take a moment and practice the Healing Exercise as you hold your baby. Relax into the space of sensitivity and mentally ask your baby what is needed. Listen to your intuition. Check with your doctor if you sense discomfort that needs attention.

- Take some time to record your feelings and evaluate your mental, physical, and spiritual states. When can you schedule, even for a few minutes daily, some of the techniques for exercise, meditation, and relaxation?

- Are you getting the support you need from your partner, family, and community? These people cannot read your mind, so make your needs known.

- If you are a single mom, or if it is not possible to get support, it is even more important for you to stay relaxed. Investigate parenting support in your local community if you feel overwhelmed.

8 Perimenopause and Menopause

Yesterday is already a dream,
And tomorrow is only a vision;
But today, well lived,
Makes every yesterday a dream of happiness
And every tomorrow a vision of hope.

—ANONYMOUS

Menopause is changing the face of medicine. Each day approximately 4,000 American women turn fifty, transitioning into the years of wisdom. There were more than 40 million menopausal women in the year 2001, and at least 25 million more women will become menopausal within the next ten years. As modern women pass through this transition into the years of wisdom, they are changing the face of medicine and the mores of Western culture.

As recently as a few decades ago, there were no birth control pills, abortion was a criminal offense, there were no home tests for ovulation and pregnancy, and infertility treatment was primitive. A woman had little control over her body during her reproductive years and even less control over her destiny as she entered perimenopause and menopause.

Women have made tremendous social and political strides since then, gaining both more choices and a louder voice. Women are living longer, healthier lives and are participating more actively in their health care. As such, women are looking for a deeper understanding of menopause as well as better options to help them through the transition. Women's groups, classes, and books on menopause and alternative healing options—including herbal therapies and the mind/body therapies of yoga and meditation—are attracting discerning women as they reach out to create community, care for their health, and empower themselves.

Women understand menopause to be a natural transition, and increasing numbers of women are questioning the automatic prescription of estrogen and hormone replacement therapy (HRT) at the first sign of changing hormone levels. After years of ignorning women in medical studies, scientists and doctors are now working hard to catch up and determine the effects of medications such as HRT. However, the results of some of these recently completed studies are not clear and are sometimes conflicting and confusing.

For those who look for the deeper meaning of menopause and desire a natural transition, yoga has much to offer. The teachings in Kundalini Yoga are empowering, natural, and nonjudgmental. Women are encouraged to find the best therapy for their transition: Some women may need supportive hormone therapies, while other women may choose a totally "natural" route. Whatever your choice, practicing yoga will always bring deep and lasting benefits.

As with all transitions in a woman's life, the yogini takes her entire life into consideration as she works through perimenopause and menopause. Consider menopause as the culmination the energies you have expended over the years. The energy that fueled menstruation, maturation, childbearing, and career, as well as all the knowledge and wisdom gained from these experiences, is reaching a critical mass at the time of menopause. As your hormones shift, your entire life shifts onto a new stage of power and projection. You can see the past, frame it, share it, and teach it. In your professional life, with your family, and in your community, you become the experienced one, the advisor, the guide. You sit on the throne of your royalty, presence, and intuition; you project with your thoughts and manifest your projects for the good of all. This is the yogic perspective of the menopausal transition.

Your day-to-day experience, however, may be quite different! You may feel mentally, physically, and spiritually challenged. Your energy levels can vacillate, and you may have difficulty sleeping. Your periods change, and the time you spend waiting for them may feel like a million years of irritability. You may feel that you see everything, finally, clearly—and you may be shocked! Women often ask themselves many questions during menopause, such as, "Is this my life?" and "What happened?" and "Why does this culture seem so ridiculous?" You may experience acute feelings of grief, elation, hope, or despair. It is common to be afraid of and depressed over the thought of aging. Yet in your cellular memories, you know the ancient symbol of the mature woman is the spiritual apex, the soothsayer, and the embodiment of compassion and intuition. Why is the menopausal experience such a paradox?

Many women report the menopausal transition to be the strongest transformation of their lives. What was said earlier about your throne of royalty and intuition is true. The brilliance of your presence is real. The polarizing feelings of this transition are accurate. Menopause can be a difficult transition because we are immersed in a culture that is superficial and encourages us to search outside of ourselves for happiness, acceptance, and beauty. From this shallow and cosmetic perspective, menopause can appear to be a physical hassle and a dreaded sign of loss of youth. The conscious menopausal woman, however, has the opportunity to reject cultural illusions and embrace both health and meaning.

Perimenopause, the years (within ten) leading up to your menopause, can be a time to see the truth, to really wake up! When the yogis say that yoga "keeps you young," they mean that through the practice of the kriyas, meditations, and pranayama, you can energize your glands and activate your awareness in order to feel the juiciness of life—the prana, or the kundalini. Youth to the yogini is the internal process of awakening your awareness to be present in each moment as a new experience in time and space. Through your heightened awareness, you can see reality; you can channel your intelligence and manifest it in the world. It is actually easier to experience this awareness as you grow older, even though your body may not be as strong. The power of millions of women in menopause can begin to transform our society into a more compassionate one of reality and respect.

We are indeed on the cusp of a new age, the Aquarian Age. According to the teachings of Yogi Bhajan and many sages and philosophers, this age will bring more polarity—more war and more peace—and a need to process your experience through your sensory self, as there are just too much data to sort through.

The Experience of Menopause

Each woman experiences the physical, emotional, and spiritual shifts during menopause differently. As your body cycles toward a new, lower level of estrogen, you may experience hot flashes, sleeplessness, and irritability, as well as unexpected bursts of energy. How you experience this physical transition is rooted in your genetics, your lifelong habits of exercise and diet, and your attitude. The goal is to stay steady through the changes by using the three elements of diet, exercise, and yoga, plus meditation and a spiritual attitude. (Later in the chapter you'll find recommended foods, supplements, and herbs for menopause.) Some women also find it best to choose a doctor or alternative therapist to help guide them through their menopausal years.

From the perspective of Kundalini Yoga, a woman's prescription for easing the symptoms of menopause is to exercise enough to sweat and to socialize with women friends enough to laugh every day. Rigorous exercising to the point of sweating, especially exercise that targets your liver and adrenal glands, will help stimulate your entire glandular system and help you maintain the best hormonal balance possible. Aerobic exercise will also keep your heart healthy. Weight-bearing exercises, such as walking and yoga, can help maintain bone mass. Laughing, too, is also a powerful medicine. Laughing releases the fear that tightens your diaphragm muscles and constricts your breathing. Laughing can relax you on all levels. It stimulates your seventh sense—your sense of humor! Laughter uplifts your spirits.

Meditation and breathing exercises can also help with perimenopausal discomfort. Long, Deep Breathing and Alternate Nostril Breathing serve to calm your mind and give you the perspective you need to withstand any physical chaos (see Chapter 1 to review these two techniques). Your spiritual and mental outlook and your ability to find meaning in your life may be the difference between feeling isolated and feeling empowered. At this time, some women begin a spiritual quest that culminates in a clearer understanding of themselves and their world. This is both an ancient and modern experience. To navigate through the menopause years, you need to use your internal compass—your intuition.

Once perimenopause is over and you no longer ovulate, your Moon Centers continue to cycle in the same sequence as they did when you were in your mother's womb. Your creativity is enhanced, and there may be a new quality to your intuition and sensitivity. This transition can be generally expressed as a move from the second chakra to the sixth, from relationship to leadership, from reason to intuition.

Although your sexual drive may lessen during perimenopause and menopause, it often returns when your body becomes used to your new chemical/hormonal status. As both men and women age, they actually become more alike in their hormonal makeup, with spiritual energies moving toward the higher chakras. As a result of these chemical, hormonal, and energy shifts, and given that sexuality begins in the upper glands and chakras, sex can be an even deeper and more universal experience. In Chapter 6 you'll find examples of yogic guidance for increasing sexual intimacy. If your libido is low, practicing the Venus Kriyas can bring both you and your partner's energies toward the upper chakras and increase your desire for sex.

Modern medicine is moving forward with antidotes for the physical discomforts of menopause. Depending on your past health or genetics, you may have symptoms that are so extreme that you need the support of hormone therapies. Don't judge yourself or others on this basis. Once you feel balanced, evaluate your life again. With a doctor's support, begin an exercise program, adjust your diet, meditate, and relax. Use your intelligence to make the best decisions regarding your well-being.

In addition to all these physical changes, as many as half of the women in menopause say they experience some degree of depression. Time alone may be enough for some women to transition through these feelings. Others may benefit from changes in diet, exercise, hormones, herbs, or supplements. If you have feelings of despair, are consistently unable to sleep, or if you have little interest in food or sex, you may be depressed. Your doctor and other health-care professionals can help you determine what extra support you may need to manage your feelings during this time of transition.

Sisterhood is essential for women and has always been a strong foundation for healing on every level. Traditionally, when women do not find what they need from conventional medicine, they begin to work together, to hold classes, write books, and interview each other regarding menopause. This camaraderie and communication is helpful to all women. Women do not need to stay silent, to whisper about menopause. The stresses of elderly parents, illness, and growing children can feel overwhelming, and the support of other women can bring great comfort and emotional release. The greater community of women is organizing itself; you can join with others in a class, or you can talk one-on-one with a sympathetic friend. Keep communicating, and try taking a yoga class or joining a meditation group. (If there are no classes near you, try looking on the Internet for other options.) Remind yourself that menopause is natural and that you can empower yourself with the best of ancient and modern approaches.

Perimenopause and Menopause | DR.'S NOTES

Menopause is not a silent passage anymore. As baby boomers age, they increasingly are finding themselves just as proud of reaching and thriving in menopause as they are of every other phase of their lives. And with good reason! If a woman reaches age fifty without contracting heart disease or cancer, she can expect to live to be ninety-two. One-third of a woman's lifetime is spent in menopause. That's great news for the more than 4,000 American women who reach age fifty each day. Knowing that menopause is just one more transition in a rich and full life allows a woman to stop asking the question "How do I stop aging?" and begin asking the question "How do I remain graceful throughout life's challenges?"

UNDERSTANDING THE LINGO

Menopause is derived from two Greek words meaning "month" and "cessation." It is not defined by an age, but by an event. Having a *hysterectomy* (surgical removal of the uterus) will also stop menstruation, but it does not cause menopause unless the ovaries are also removed (called an *oophorectomy*). Whether the ovaries simply cease making enough estrogen to create a menstrual cycle (natural or spontaneous menopause), are removed by surgery (surgical menopause), or destroyed by radiation treatments, chemotherapy, or some other means (induced menopause), a woman's last menstrual period defines menopause. The tricky part about defining menopause is that you must wait one full year after your last period to confirm the diagnosis and make certain it's not just an irregular period.

The average age of natural menopause is 51.4 years in the United States (in a range of 40–55 years of age). *Premature menopause* is the term given to menopause occurring before age 40 (this occurs in about 2 percent of women). *Perimenopause* means, literally, "around menopause" and refers to the months and years (up to ten) leading up to menopause, plus one year after the last menstrual period. In 1990 there were an estimated 28.7 million women older than fifty-five in the United States. By 2000 that number had increased to 31.2 million, and by 2020 the projected number of women who will be in menopause is 45.9 million.

THE SIGNS AND THE SYMPTOMS

Perimenopause and menopause are times of change—tremendous change. Not a change into another person but into another phase of life. Not from health to disease but from one natural state to another. And, as it is with every change, it is a time of transition.

Experiencing perimenopause and menopause is a lot like going through puberty–only in reverse! Like puberty, perimenopause and menopause are also times of erratic estrogen and progesterone levels. When a woman reaches age thirty-eight or so, eggs are lost from the ovaries at an accelerated rate, leaving a woman at age forty with 5,000–10,000 eggs out of the 400,000 eggs she was born with. When she is fifty-one, all of these remaining eggs are usually gone and with them the surrounding cells that produce most of the body's estrogen and progesterone. During this time, the exquisitely coordinated hormones of reproduction begin to lose their ability to work together with precision, causing changes in menstrual cycle patterns, mood, sleep, concentration, sexual desires, breast firmness, and a changing body image. Brain receptors that help reduce anxiety no longer receive steady amounts of progesterone, leaving some women feeling anxious or depressed. Fluctuating levels of estrogen and progesterone also cause an imbalance in the brain's thermostat, interrupting the autonomic nervous system and creating sudden changes in skin temperature.

These changes result in the most common reason for which a woman in menopause seeks medical attention—hot flashes.

Like puberty, there is no blueprint for menopause. Each woman is an individual; it's no wonder there are such extreme differences in women who are going through perimenopause and menopause. Some women sail through, while others are greatly affected. But all are aware that they are experiencing a transition. The good news is that, like the symptoms of puberty, those of menopause end, and allow one's true self to reemerge. Common symptoms of perimenopause include:

- Hot flashes

- Insomnia

- Menstrual cycle irregularities

- Memory problems (usually caused by disturbed sleep)

- Vaginal dryness

- Lower sexual desire

- Anxiety

- Mood swings

COPING WITH SYMPTOMS

The fact that estrogen is responsible for breast development, body contour, and many distinctly feminine traits makes it a truism that estrogen contributes to "shaping" a woman. Estrogen levels are exceedingly low during the first decade of a woman's life, when boys and girls are more similar than different. Levels then start to rise, and for three decades, approximately ten to forty times more estrogen flows through a woman's veins to every part of her body—from her head to her toes. Then follows a decade of declining estrogen levels until once again estrogen drops to prepubertal amounts. Because estrogen levels fluctuate throughout a woman's lifetime, from very low to very high, it is difficult to accept that one level is more normal than another or that a lower level is a deficiency.

Many women wonder if hormone replacement therapy (HRT) is the best way to deal with the onset of menopause and its many symptoms. And while everyone agrees that menopause is a time of lower estrogen levels, there is a lively controversy surrounding HRT's benefits and risks. How much estrogen your body should be producing depends on the stage of life you are in. It also depends on your symptoms, medical history, family history, age, medications, and a host of other factors that every woman should discuss with her doctor. While HRT may be the answer to combating the symptoms of menopause, there are other alternatives, including diet, supplements, herbal remedies, and exercise—particularly yoga.

PERIMENOPAUSE AND BEYOND: A PRESCRIPTION FOR HEALTH

Herbal Remedies	Exercise & Yoga	Diet & Supplements
Black Cohosh: Available as tablets, capsules, and tinctures. Studies show it can help relieve hot flashes. **Evening Primrose Oil:** About 3 grams daily to help alleviate breast tenderness and hot flashes and to balance hormone levels. **Dong Quai:** A Chinese herb often used to relieve menstrual cramps and menopausal symptoms. Recent studies don't support these claims, but Chinese herbs are traditionally prescribed in combination and not alone.	**Vigorous Exercise and Laughing:** Exercise (best if done earlier in the day) helps metabolism and sleep. Can include brisk walking and selected yoga that makes you sweat. **Meditations:** Choose meditations that match your needs for balance, energy, and relaxation. If you are feeling down or processing deep feelings, get help and choose meditations that help you to release tension and process feelings. Transform emotion into devotion.	**Soy:** Contains natural estrogens. Benefits include reduction of hot flashes and vaginal dryness, promotion of bone and heart health, and possible reduction of cancer risk. Available as tofu, soy milk, tempeh, soy beans (usually $1/2$–1 cup daily), soy powder (40 grams daily), and capsules (50 mg daily) such as SoyCare. **Caloric Intake:** Reduce 50 calories daily each year after age forty to maintain weight.

Yoga can help to balance the many changes of menopause. Perimenopause and menopause are wonderful times to incorporate yoga and the yogic lifestyle into your life. By increasing the oxygen in your body and mind, and sharpening your ability to concentrate, yoga can help you achieve a sense of balance with your emotions and restore equilibrium to a body that is fluctuating enormously. As you slow your heart and respiratory rates and lower your level of stress, you will synchronize and balance your automatic nervous system. Refer to the table on page 164 and below for recommendations on how yoga and natural remedies can relieve the symptoms of perimenopause and menopause.

PERIMENOPAUSE AND BEYOND: A PRESCRIPTION FOR HEALTH		
Herbal Remedies	**Exercise & Yoga**	**Diet & Supplements**
Chasteberry (Vitex): May help with menstrual irregularities and painful breasts. Also used for PMS. Available as teas, tinctures, or 2-mg capsules twice daily. **St. John's Wort:** Nicknamed "natural Prozac" because of its beneficial effect on depression and anxiety. Available as teas, tinctures, or 300-mg capsules twice or three times daily.	**Catnaps:** Aim for 11–20 minutes for maximum rejuvenation. Best time is between 4:00 and 6:00 P.M. **Personal Needs:** Become your own personal trainer. Socialize. Maintain and care for your body, mind, and spirit.	**General Guidelines:** Eat a lighter diet with plenty of fresh fruits and vegetables, and few fried and processed foods. **Vitamin E:** Potent antioxidant that may reduce the risk of certain cancers and heart attack. High dosages may reduce hot flashes. Dosages of up to 800 mg daily have been found safe. **Calcium:** Average daily intake below 600 mg. Daily need 1,200 mg. Virtually essential to reduce the risk of osteoporosis. Best absorbed with vitamin D and small amounts of magnesium.

Sexuality and Intimacy During Menopause

As you enter perimenopause or menopause, you may notice some changes in your sexual response. Lower estrogen levels reduce vaginal lubrication, so it may take longer to be ready for intercourse because of vaginal dryness. Over-the-counter vaginal lubricants or almond oil and vitamin E supplementation can be useful to restore lubrication. It is also recommended to practice Kegel exercises. The Root Lock (see Chapter 2 for review) strengthens your pelvic floor muscles. Tightening your vaginal and pelvic floor muscles can increase your sexual pleasure and give you more bladder control. You may do Kegel exercises six times daily, in sets of ten.

Every Woman Is Unique

If declining levels of estrogen cause all the symptoms of menopause, why don't all women experience them? Scientists and researchers do not yet know the answer to this question. The yogis are careful to view the body as more than the sum of its parts, and we believe that science will eventually show this to be true. Likewise, science may show that your lifestyle, diet, spiritual well-being, and environment affect menopausal symptoms as well.

As spiritual beings in a human existence, we are constantly trying to balance the health of our physical bodies. Old age and illness in some form or other will befall us all. The yogic wisdom of living a neutral life in the timeless reality of the soul, unaffected by the polarities of young/old and sickness/health may at times seems unattainable. The time you take each day to put your life in perspective, meditate and conquer your fear, and enjoy each breath is one step toward living in a timeless, unattached manner. Many masters of yoga and other spiritual disciplines describe the journey each person makes as having profound value. Science may be discovering just now that the spiritual path has health benefits, too. Affirms Yogi Bhajan: "It's not the life that you live. It's the courage that you bring to it."

You can make certain dietary changes after forty years of age to support your transition through perimenopause and menopause. As you age, your nutritional needs change. From the yogic perspective, one of the most important aspects of diet is how much you eat.

After forty, and especially during menopause, your body needs less food. People in Western cultures typically overeat. Half of all Americans are overweight, and one-fourth are significantly overweight. If you refine your diet following these basic recommendations, you can improve your health and increase your energy level. For additional natural remedies to alleviate some of the common symptoms of menopause and all stages of life, refer to Appendix A.

Steamed Greens

Choose your favorite fresh green vegetables and steam them using fresh, clean water. Steam until the vegetables are bright green. Do not overcook them. Eat the vegetables as a light meal in the evening. You can drink the broth as a healthy tonic for your liver. If your digestion is sluggish, try a day of steamed greens to support your elimination and nurture your body.

The Woman's Drink

The following drink is said to keep a woman very healthy and help her through menopause. It is very strong and has a cleansing effect on the body. The lemon and ginger ingredients have a detoxifying effect on the liver, and the oil is supportive of your hormonal balance. Give it a try if you have a juicer (a blender will not be able to extract juice from ginger), or have the juice bar at your health food store make one for you. Remember that this is using food as medicine, so start out with a few sips and build up to a full drink over time.

> 2 oz. lemon juice
> 2 oz. ginger juice
> 1 oz. sesame oil

Mix together in a juicer and enjoy.

Soy Power!

Soy has so many nutritional and medicinal benefits that it is now considered a staple for women in perimenopause and menopause. In my book *The Soy Solution for Menopause,* I discuss specific studies that show how soy can reduce hot flashes, improve the elasticity of the blood vessels, lower cholesterol, keep bones healthy, and reduce the risk of certain cancers. Here are some soy recipes you will enjoy.

No-Egg Egg Salad

> 1 lb. firm low-fat tofu
>
> 1 large stalk celery, chopped
>
> ¼ cup onion, finely chopped
>
> ¼ cup tofu mayonnaise (available in health food stores)
>
> 1 tbsp. prepared mustard

Mash the tofu with a fork in a large bowl until it becomes crumbly. Add the celery, onion, mayonnaise, mustard, and other seasonings you enjoy; mix thoroughly. Serve on whole-grain or pita bread with sliced tomatoes and sprouts.
Serves 4.

Gilda's Kale with Tofu

The key to this recipe is in the kale preparation. Be sure to use fresh kale and chop it very finely so you can cook it in less time. This is a delicious and fast way to include kale in your diet. Each cup of cooked kale provides 94 mg of calcium, 296 mg of potassium, 9,620 IU of vitamin A, 17.3 mcg of folic acid, 53.3 mg of vitamin C, 23.4 mg of magnesium, and many other healthful nutrients.

> 2 tbsp. olive oil
>
> 3 cups kale, finely chopped
>
> ½ lb. tofu, cubed
>
> 2–3 cloves garlic, finely chopped
>
> Salt (and other seasonings you enjoy) to taste

Heat the olive oil in a skillet, add the chopped kale, tofu, and garlic; sauté until the kale is deep green and soft. Remove from heat; season to taste. Serve over pasta, rice, or alone.

These gentle exercises will help alleviate the symptoms of menopause. Practice them separately or in a sequence as a part of your yoga routine.

Walking

Whether you have been exercising your whole life or are just beginning an exercise program, walking is one of the best ways to get in shape. The motion of your body when you walk will massage your inner organs and exercise your muscles and bones. If you are just beginning to exercise, start with 20 minutes per day and work up to 3–5 miles daily.

Half-Wheel Pose

Lie on your back. Bend your knees, bringing your feet flat on the floor as close to your buttocks as is comfortable, keeping your heels about 18 inches apart. Grasp your ankles and raise your buttocks and torso off the floor, stretching your belly toward the ceiling (if you cannot grasp your ankles, place your hands by your sides, palms facing down, and use them to help you hold the posture). Hold this stretch with Long, Deep Breathing. Build up to holding this posture for up to 3 minutes. To end, slowly bring your back to the floor, and relax on your back.

Benefits This exercise helps to adjust your reproductive organs and strengthens your spine.

Liver-Cleansing Twist

Sit in Easy Pose (cross-legged). Place your right hand behind your back with the back of your hand against your lower back. Stretch your left arm up to 60 degrees from your side with your elbow straight. Hold this posture while you twist your torso left and right. Inhale to the left and exhale to the right. Continue this motion for 1–3 minutes.

Benefits This is a gentle exercise to stimulate liver cleansing.

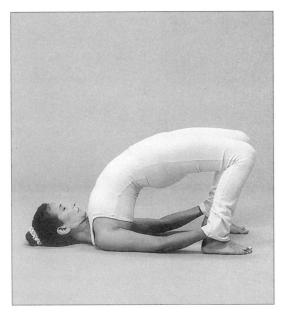

Half-Wheel Pose

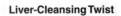

Liver-Cleansing Twist

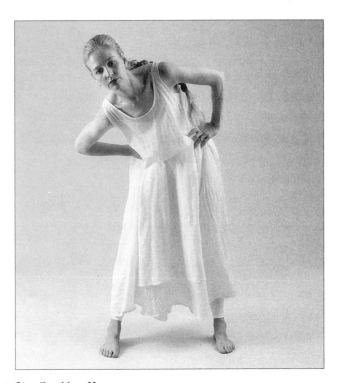

Standing Liver Massage

Standing Liver Massage

Stand on your feet with your legs about 18 inches apart. Place your hands on your hips. Begin making large circles with your upper body, stretching as you circle slowly around. Continue this circling motion for up to 11 minutes.

Benefits This liver exercise is quite healthy for you. If you can build it up to 11 minutes and eat well, you can achieve optimal liver function.

Liver-Cleansing Breath

Sit in Easy Pose. Relax your hands in your lap or in Gyan Mudra. Keeping your tongue relaxed and wide, stick your tongue out of your mouth past your lips. Close the center of your lips around your tongue, keeping the sides open as if you are smiling. Inhale and exhale slowly through the sides of your mouth. Continue for 1–3 minutes.

Exercise Set for Glandular Strength and Liver Health

Your liver, spleen, and pancreas collect the toxins resulting from your diet and pollution. When these organs become full of toxins, your blood cannot be filtered properly. Efficient liver function is important during menopause because the liver helps to normalize the level of hormones in the blood. The exercises that follow are considered an excellent tonic for these organs and glands.

1. **Pumping Your Navel Point.** Sit in Easy Pose with your spine straight. Inhale slowly, taking a full 5 seconds to complete your inhalation. Exhale slowly, taking a full 5 seconds to complete your exhalation. Hold your breath out for 15 seconds while you pump your navel point in and out in a steady rhythm. (Really pull it up high and then push it out!) Continue for 5 minutes. To end, inhale and suspend your breath briefly. Exhale and relax.

2. **Liver Leg Lift.** Lie on your back, with your legs straight and ankles together. Inhale, raise your legs 60 degrees from the floor, and hold this position for 15 seconds. Exhale as you bring your knees to your

chest, grabbing your knees with your hands to hold them close to your chest. Hold this position with your breath out for 15 seconds. Inhale, return your legs to the 60-degree position, and hold for 15 seconds. Exhale, lower your legs to the floor, and hold 15 seconds. Repeat this sequence eight times. Relax for 5 minutes.

This exercise sequence can be rigorous. Be sure to keep pressing your lower spine into the floor as you hold your legs out. Start by holding the breath for 5–10 seconds or do a few repetitions until you can build up to 15 seconds.

Benefits This kriya will bring new circulation to your liver, spleen, and adrenals. It's worth the effort!

3. *Tiger Pose.* Sit on your right heel and extend your left leg straight behind you with no bend in the knee. Let your head fall back so your back is arched to its maximum. Bend your arms with your elbows as close to your sides as possible, hands at shoulder height, palms facing the sky. Hold for 5 minutes with Long, Deep Breathing. Change sides (sitting on left heel, right leg extended) and continue for 5 minutes (a total of 10 minutes maximum).

Benefits This exercise is highly recommended for perimenopausal women. It can be practiced regularly and on its own to achieve many benefits. This exercise massages your liver, reproductive organs, kidneys, and adrenals. Build up to 5 minutes with practice. You will gain strength and help your body to maintain the proper hormonal balance through doing this exercise.

4. *Leg Raises.* Lie on your back with your feet 3 feet apart, arms at your sides, about 3 feet away from your body. With your arms and legs straight, raise them 2 feet from the floor. Use deep, powerful breathing. Hold this posture until your body begins to shake. Make sure you keep your abdominal muscles tight and your lower back pressing toward the floor, to avoid putting undue stress on your back. Relax.

Benefits This exercise stimulates your circulation after the massaging of your organs in the previous exercise. It can make you sweat and help strengthen your nervous system and your lower back.

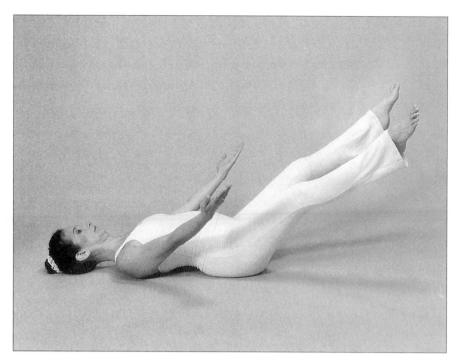

Liver Leg Lift

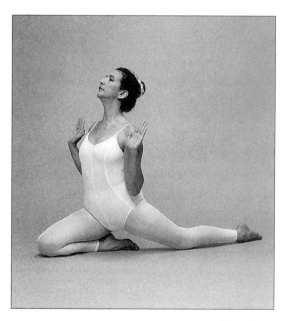

Tiger Pose

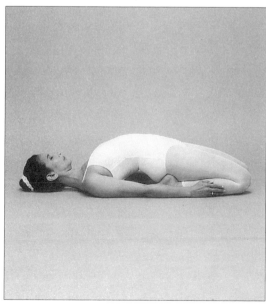

Body Stretch in Rock Pose

5. **Body Stretch in Rock Pose.** Sit either on your heels, in Half-Lotus, or in Lotus position. Lie flat on your back, arms at your sides, and relax in this position with Long, Deep Breathing. After 3 minutes, gently and gracefully stretch your legs out straight and relax.

Benefits This exercise will help your digestion and increase your flexibility. Recommended for advanced yoginis.

6. **Relax.** Take time to relax on your back for up to 11 minutes. Follow with a meditation.

Exercise Set for Strength and Humor

This kriya is also recommended for women going through menopuase. It is also a set of exercises that stimulates liver function.

1. **Hip Stretch.** Sitting in Easy Pose, bring the soles of your feet together. Hold on to your feet and bend forward at your waist, bringing your head toward your feet. Hold this position with Long, Deep Breathing for 3–5 minutes. To end, inhale, rise up, and relax.

2. **Triangle Pose.** Start by crouching on your hands and knees. Curl your toes under and press your palms into the floor as you raise your tailbone toward the ceiling, forming the shape of a triangle with your body. Allow your head to relax down between your elbows and stretch the tailbone up and your heels to the floor. Hold this posture for 3–5 minutes with Long, Deep Breathing.

3. **Buttocks Kicks.** Still in Triangle Pose, begin alternately kicking your buttocks with your heels. (First kick with the left leg, then with the right.) Continue steadily for 3–5 minutes. To end, relax and release the pose.

4. **Laughing.** Sit in Easy Pose. Bring your head back and laugh out loud. Fake it until you make it if you have to, but show your teeth and laugh! Continue laughing for 1 minute and then relax.

Benefits Laughing releases tension and is comforting to your heart. Do not underestimate the power of laughter.

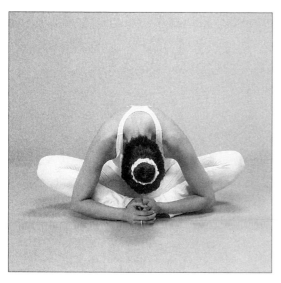

Hip Stretch

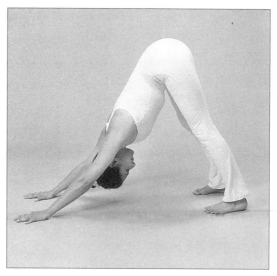

Triangle Pose

5. ***Shifting Your Waist.*** Sit in Rock Pose (on your heels) and rest your hands on your thighs. Move your waist 6 inches to the left and then 6 inches to the right. Continue this movement for 3–5 minutes.

Benefits This exercise stimulates your digestive system.

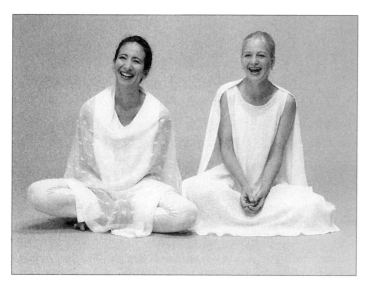

Laughing

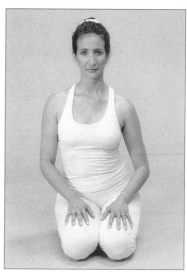

Shifting Your Waist

6. ***Chanting* Wha Hay Guroo.** Sit in Easy Pose. Relax your hands in Gyan Mudra, index finger and thumb coming together in a circle, wrists resting on your knees. Close your eyes and focus on your brow point. Softly and calmly chant the mantra *Wha Hay Guroo* (pronounced *wha-hey-goo-roo*). Continue chanting for 3–11 minutes.

Benefits After exercising strenuously, this meditation will help you deeply relax and heal.

7. ***Relax.*** Enjoy the benefits of this kriya.

Yoga Set for Emotional Balance

1. ***Miracle Bend.*** Assume a standing position. Place your knees and heels together with your feet flat on the floor and angled out to 45 degrees for balance. Raise your arms straight over your head with your palms facing forward (you can hook your thumbs together to help hold up your arms). Keep your legs straight but avoid locking your knee joints. Stretch up and bend back 20 degrees. Your head, spine, and arms should form an unbroken curve, with your arms remaining in line with your ears. You may shake in this posture, but do your best to keep up and stretch. Hold this stretch gently with Long, Deep Breathing for 2 minutes.

Benefits Called the "miracle bend," this exercise is said to "bend the negativity out of the human being" (Yogi Bhajan). It will adjust your navel point, balancing your energy and turning anger into calmness.

2. ***Pumping the Navel Point.*** From the above position, bend forward very slowly, keeping your arms straight and close to your ears. Let your torso and your arms hang to the floor. Inhale and suspend your breath in, pumping your belly in and out. Then exhale, hold the breath out, and pump your belly in and out again. Continue the sequence of holding the breath in and out and pumping your belly for 2 minutes. To end, relax your breath and slowly stand up and relax.

Benefits Together with the preceding exercise, this exercise works to help alleviate feelings of insecurity.

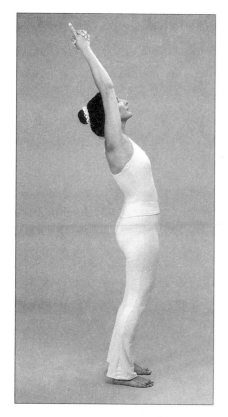

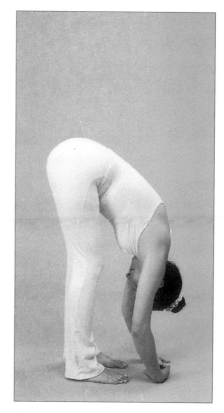

Miracle Bend   **Pumping the Navel Point**

3. ***Hip Rotation.*** Return to a standing position. Spread your legs apart so your feet are as far apart as you can comfortably hold them without losing your balance. Bend your elbows and hold your upper arms by your side with your forearms parallel to the floor. Begin to rotate your hips in large circles, as large as you can, at a moderate pace. The direction can be either clockwise or counterclockwise. Continue rotating your hips in this way for 2 minutes. Relax.

Benefits This exercise works on the lower back and hips. It can awaken in you a fearless spirit! This is a common exercise in the military and is done before battle, to loosen up.

4. ***Arm Rotation.*** Place your legs and feet in the same position as in the previous exercise. Hold your arms straight out from your body. Begin a backward rotation of your arms, with one arm rotating clockwise

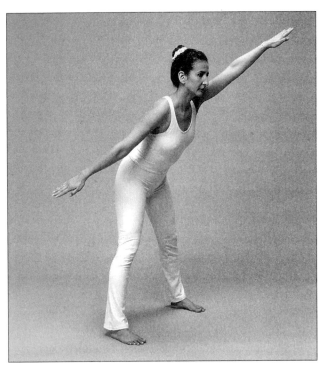

Arm Rotation

and the other rotating counterclockwise. As you rotate your arms, keep them at least 30 degrees away from your body. Rotate your arms at one rotation per second. While you rotate your arms in this way, bend forward halfway toward the floor, then straighten up and bend backward halfway to your maximum stretch. Each cycle of bending forward, straightening, bending back, and straightening takes 15 seconds. Continue this exercise for 1½ minutes. To end the exercise, stand straight up and relax.

Benefits This exercise may seem like a brain-teaser! Rotating your arms in different directions takes concentration and coordination. This exercise increases stamina and clear thinking, and can help prevent an early menopause.

5. **Relax.** Relax on your back with your spine in alignment and your arms relaxed by your side with your palms facing upward. You must relax for 10 minutes after this exercise set to receive its full effects and benefits.

1. Sit in Easy Pose or in a chair with your feet flat on the floor. Hold your forearms straight out in front of your body parallel to the floor with your elbows bent close to your body, near your rib cage. Place your right palm facing down toward the earth, and your left palm facing up toward the sky. Begin a segmented breath, inhaling in eight equal segments and exhaling in eight equal segments. On each segment of your breath, alternately move your hands and forearms up and down six to eight inches. As one hand moves up, the other moves down, as if you are bouncing a ball. Breathe powerfully as you continue this breath and movement sequence for 9 minutes. You can use the sound of your breath as your mantra or mentally chant *Saa Taa Naa Maa* twice on each inhalation and twice on each exhalation. Each syllable goes with one breath segment. Continue for 9 minutes.

2. Keep both hands and forearms parallel to the floor. Close your eyes and focus on the center of your chin. Allow your body to remain still and heal itself. Quiet your mind and relax your breath for 6 minutes.

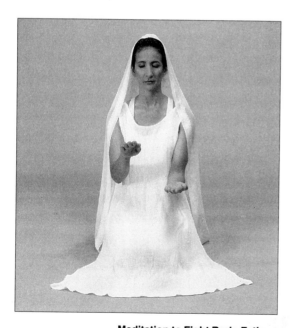

Meditation to Fight Brain Fatigue

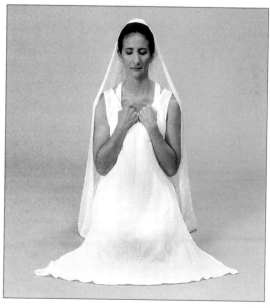

Meditation to Fight Brain Fatigue—(ending)

3. To end this three-part meditation, inhale deeply and suspend your breath while you make your hands into fists and press them forcefully against your chest for 15 seconds. Exhale. Inhale deeply again and suspend your breath while you press your fists against your navel point for 15 seconds. Exhale. Inhale deeply once more and suspend your breath while you bend your elbows and hold your fists near your shoulders, pressing your arms forcefully against your rib cage for 15 seconds. Exhale and relax.

Benefits This meditation is excellent for relaxing your brain and helping you to focus and calm your mind. It can help balance the hemispheres of your brain, and relieve the imbalance you may feel as a result of hormonal changes. This meditation has a positive effect also on your liver, navel point, spleen, and lymphatic system.

Alternate Nostril Breathing

Sit in Easy Pose or in a chair with your feet flat on the floor. Hold your left hand in Gyan Mudra, resting on your knee. Use your right thumb to close your right nostril as you inhale through your left nostril. When you reach a full inhalation, close your left nostril with your right index finger and remove your thumb to open your right nostril. Exhale through your right nostril. When you reach a complete exhalation, inhale through your right nostril. At your full inhalation point, switch from your index finger to your thumb (covering your right nostril) and exhale through your left nostril. Continue this sequence:

> Inhale left, exhale right.
> Inhale right, exhale left.
> Inhale left, exhale right.

Continue this breath sequence, consciously taking long, deep breaths. Keep your breath smooth without straining. You can concentrate on the sound of your breath or the mantra *Sat* on the inhalation and *Naam* on the exhalation. Meditate in this manner for 3–31 minutes.

Benefits Alternate Nostril Breathing is a basic and beautiful way to bring balance to the hemispheres of your brain, which can be especially helpful

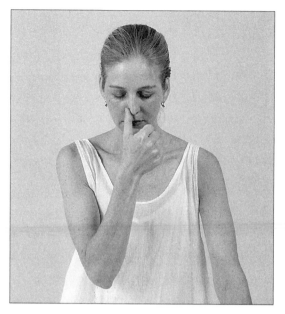

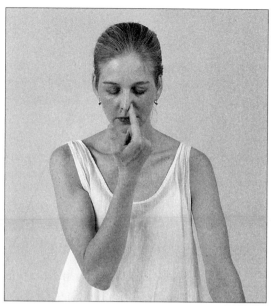

Alternate Nostril Breathing (right nostril)

Alternate Nostril Breathing (left nostril)

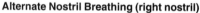

during menopause. It is a powerful tonic for your nervous and glandular systems and is highly recommended for practice at all stages of life.

Meditation to Release Stress

This meditation is especially beneficial for releasing stress related to family relationships. Sit in Easy Pose or in a chair with your feet flat on the floor. Place your hands together, palms facing each other in front of your chest area. Touch the fingertips and thumb tips of your right hand to the fingertips and thumb tips of your left hand, forming a triangle with your hands while your thumbs point toward your chest. (There is a space between the palms of your right and left hands.) Point your fingers upward. Focus your eyes on the tip of your nose and breathe four times per minute. Inhale for 5 seconds, suspend your

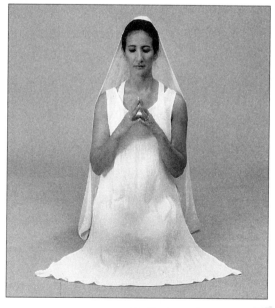

Meditation to Release Stress

breath for 5 seconds, and exhale for 5 seconds. Continue for 11 minutes or until you feel relief from the stress.

Grace of God Meditation

This meditation is described in Chapter 5. During menopause, you can practice it three times a day to remind your body, mind, and soul of your infinite and divine nature. Practiced regularly, the effects of this meditation will be lasting.

DR.'S NOTES

Breathing and the Brain

As you have learned, Pranayama, or breathing exercise, is a major component of Kundalini Yoga. Yoga teachers often describe the powerful changes that breathing patterns can create, particularly in brain activity. The brain's ability to perform certain functions is centered in the right or the left half. The right side, for instance, is involved with spatial relationships, the left with verbal skills and understanding. In a recent study, men and women were asked to breathe through their right or left nostril (as in alternate nostril breathing), or to use breathing awareness through both nostrils. When the male subjects breathed through the left nostril, there was a beneficial effect on the left (verbal) side of the brain. Those breathing through the right nostril improved in spatial abilities. The women in the study reported different effects: those breathing through the left nostril improved their right (spatial) brain function, while their verbal function was not affected. Yogic breathing and meditation can help bring oxygen to the frontal cortex and anterior cingulated gyri, and to temporal and parietal areas of the brain, and can help slow metabolism and help send energy to areas of the brain where it is most needed.

Gentle Yoga for Perimenopause

Full-body self-massage and cold shower hydrotherapy (not when menstruating) in the morning or at any time of day when you have time for self-healing therapies.

1. Tune in.

2. Spinal Flex and Spinal Twist, twenty-six times each.

3. Liver Cleansing Breath for 1–3 minutes.

4. Liver Cleansing Twist, twenty-six times.

5. Half-Wheel with Long, Deep Breathing for 1–3 minutes.

6. Alternate Nostril Breathing for 7–11 minutes.

7. Relax for 11 minutes.

Add 15–30 minutes of walking daily to this gentle yoga workout. Work up to being comfortable with walking briskly for 30 minutes. If you cannot walk, add another exercise (e.g., cycling on an exercise bike, gardening, etc.) that you can do until you sweat. Also practice until you can flex your spine gently for 3 minutes.

Challenging Yoga for Perimenopause

In addition to this routine, practice full-body self-massage and cold shower hydrotherapy (not when menstruating) in the morning or at any time of day when you have time for self-healing therapies.

1. Tune in.

2. Breath of Fire for 1–3 minutes.

3. Choose one of these yoga sets from the chapter: Exercise Set for Strength and Humor, Exercise Set for Emotional Balance, or Exercise Set for Glandular Strength and Liver Health.

4. Relax.

5. Alternate Nostril Breathing for 7–31 minutes.

6. Relax.

For a full workout, add brisk walking to this yoga routine. You can do the Alternate Nostril Breathing separate from the yoga set (i.e., at another time of day), but for best results, do the entire practice. The exercise sets prepare you for experiencing the depth of the Alternate Nostril Breathing. Add the Grace of God Meditation when you feel particularly challenged by either your physical symptoms or the demands of your life. (Repeating this meditation twice daily, morning and night, yields excellent results.)

QUESTIONS FOR FURTHER GROWTH

- Chart your monthly menstrual cycle. In perimenopause, your periods can become irregular. In addition, the sensations you feel at this time are the result of your hormonal fluctuations. Are you in perimenopause?

- Evaluate your diet, mental attitude (positive, negative, meditative, relaxed), and physical activity. Keep a journal of these three aspects for a week. Review the section on diet for perimenopause in Chapter 9. Based on your findings, what is most important for you to adjust first—meal times, diet, or attitude?

- Choose a yoga routine, exercise routine, meditation practice, and relaxation technique to keep yourself balanced.

- When was the last time you really laughed?

- How do you feel about your body? Full-body self-massage is a helpful and gentle way to learn to appreciate and love your body.

- What are your beliefs and attitudes about aging?

Yoga for the Menopausal Woman

After you have completed ovulating and have not had a menstrual cycle for 12 months, you are considered to be in menopause. During this phase of life, the world is open to you—and it is a time of refinement. Exercise at your own level, enjoying all the practices that are available to you. You can tailor your yoga program to your needs. If you want to increase your digestive fire, relax your emotions, release negativity, and empower your spirit, find the different combinations of exercise sets and meditations that work for you. Create a routine that keeps your bones, heart, body, mind, and spirit strong. Practice your routine or meditation for 40 days, and really take the time to experience the depth of that practice before trying another technique. A sample routine is listed next. Enjoy!

Yoga for Accepting Change and Energizing Your Body

1. Tune in.

2. Breath of Fire for 1–3 minutes.

3. Basic Spinal Energy Series with Sat Kriya.

4. Forward Bend.

5. Bow Pose.

6. Kirtan Kriya.

7. Relax for 11 minutes.

QUESTIONS FOR FURTHER GROWTH

• Review the lessons you have learned in your life. How can you share this wisdom with others—family, friends, community— through the arts?

- Is your creativity being expressed to its fullest? What project could you do to increase your satisfaction regarding your self-expression?

- As a woman ages, her ability to manifest through intuition and being rather than through doing is stronger. Are you letting your intuition work for you?

- In menopause, women sometimes confront nagging physical or emotional wounds that they have avoided working through. What do you need to heal? What support do you need to accomplish this healing?

Food and Digestion

You must eat what you can digest. You must eat what you can hold. And if anything has put a shadow on you, if it makes you feel that you are getting lower in grade, or not feeling good, it's better to avoid that situation.

—Yogi Bhajan

Our bodies are composed of billions of cells, each a living organism that depends on the food we eat for fuel and energy. Foods that cannot be digested or that contain no nutritional value require our bodies to use energy to eliminate them with little or no gain. Foods eaten in excess of our needs put additional stress on our digestive system and can cause us to gain weight. Some staples in the modern American diet are actually harmful! To support a healthy lifestyle, it is important to maintain a diet of fresh, nutritious, natural foods that provide the fuel our cells need for health and energy.

Choosing the right foods is difficult for many of us. Several guidelines used by the yogis can help you make these choices. The first, most basic choice is to eat nutritious foods that give the body fuel, energy, and strength. Fresh fruits, vegetables, soy, and legumes are good examples; junk foods and highly processed foods, of course, are not. Whenever possible, choose organic goods, which are the purest food sources available today. One alternative is to eat "sustaining" foods that combine nutritious content, texture, taste, and aroma. Preparing food with these four components in mind sustains and heals you.

The yogis also say to eat plenty of Sun foods, Ground foods, and Earth foods. Sun foods, mostly fruits, grow more than 3 feet above the ground and absorb maximum energy from the sun. Ground foods grow within 3 feet above the ground and are very cleansing because of their fiber content and nutritious value (for instance, rice, beans, and leafy vegetables). Earth foods, such as garlic, onion, and ginger, grow below the ground and have healing properties. Many Earth foods are actually ancient forms of medicine and are commonly sold as over-the-counter remedies.

Each of these food types creates certain effects on your body and mind. Sun foods keep the body light and etheric. Ground foods supply the basics of a healthy diet and help the body and mind feel steady and focused. Earth foods are used for their healing properties and can be stimulating and helpful in providing energy and cleansing the body of toxins. Choosing a combination of Sun, Ground, and Earth foods makes for a well-balanced diet that will enhance your life.

You can also categorize foods as Sattvic, Rajasic, or Tamasic, based on their interaction with the body. Sattvic foods are easily digested (fruits, steamed vegetables, and some legumes, such as lentils or mung beans). Rajasic foods stimulate your body (onions, garlic, and ginger). Tamasic foods deplete your energy, require prolonged digestion, and make you feel heavy (animal protein, deep-fried foods, highly saturated fatty foods). Because you are creating your future with every bite of food you eat, choose foods that match the kinds of energy you need and that support your spiritual projection. A good yogic diet would include mostly Sattvic foods, with some Rajasic foods to help you meet the challenges of your day. Limit or avoid Tamasic foods.

What, When, and How You Eat

It may be helpful to take some time to try to understand your personal eating style—what you eat, when you eat, and how you eat it. Because food is a basic form of nurturing, the emotional issues you face may be reflected in the way you eat. If you either undereat or overeat as a way of coping with emotional stress, it may be necessary to reevaluate your relationship with food, and perhaps visit a nutritionist for input. In the meantime, consider the yogic point of view on what, when, and how to eat.

What to Eat

The beginning section of this chapter offers the best guidelines for what to eat. In addition to these guidelines, avoid alcohol, excess coffee, caffeinated teas (except green teas), soft drinks, refined sugars and carbohydrates, and excess salt. Two simple dietary additions can add some quick yogic benefits: eggplant, which is regarded as a powerful healing food for women, and 1 2 tablespoons daily of a cold-pressed oil such as flaxseed, almond, or sesame. Natural cold-pressed oils can help balance your hormone levels and improve digestion.

When to Eat

Digestion is most efficient midday, so lunch is the sensible time for you to have your main meal. If you eat the bulk of your calories between 11:00 A.M. and 2:00 P.M., you will have plenty of energy to go through the day and fuel your activities. Eat a snack of raisins and a few nuts or a banana at about 4:00 P.M. to keep your minerals and sugar balanced. As sunset approaches, eat a light meal of easily digestible food. Steamed vegetables or light vegetable salads are good choices for an evening meal.

It is best not to eat after sunset. When the sun sets, your body slows down and begins to prepare for rest. Do not eat after 7:00 P.M. or 3 hours before bed. Many women suffer from heartburn and acid reflux, which makes it impossible to lie flat without heartburn and may cause sleep disturbances. A woman may find relief from her symptoms by adjusting her diet and the timing of her meals.

In short, try this schedule of eating: a light liquid meal for breakfast and midafternoon (such as the Ms. Whiz recipe later in this chapter), a solid meal midday, and a light, solid meal for dinner that is easily digestible, such as steamed vegetables and tofu or another light protein. This schedule can keep your energy and sugar level constant, and helps prevent the urge to snack.

How to Eat

Be conscious of your environment while eating. Try not to eat while watching TV or working, and give yourself a few moments after eating to "settle" your food rather than jump up immediately from the table. If you pay attention to your body as you are eating, you can stop when you feel full. Listen to the signals your body is sending you—don't continue to eat beyond the first sensation of being full. Follow this general rule: Make two fists of your hands and hold them next to each other in front of your stomach. This is the *total* amount of food you should have in your stomach at any one time. The yogic prescription for filling your stomach is one-third food, one-third water, and one-third space for digestion.

Transit Time

In addition to when you eat, it is important how long food stays in your system. This is called *transit time,* and implies how efficiently your system digests and absorbs your food. For women, the recommended estimated transit time is 12–18 hours. This means that you can eliminate the wastes of whatever you eat within 12–18 hours of eating. This is one reason why many yogis are vegetarians. The transit time for meat is up to 72 hours! The yogini wants all of her energy to go toward realizing her highest potential, not toward inefficient digestion. As you become more sensitive to your digestive process, you will notice the transit time of the foods you eat.

Any difficulty you have with elimination will affect your health and mood. Each time you eat, you stimulate your digestion to absorb new energy and eliminate waste. For this reason, the yogis believe that normal elimination occurs two to three times a day, in the morning and typically after you eat. If you are not eliminating daily, include lots of steamed green vegetables in your diet and avoid processed foods and heavy fats until your digestion is back on track.

Nutritional Needs and the Life Cycle

Throughout your life your body is constantly changing. It's not surprising that at each stage of your life cycle, your nutritional needs change as well. Here are some nutritional guidelines to keep in mind during each stage. For further information on vitamin and mineral supplementation for each of these stages, see Appendix B.

Teenagers

You can do a great deal in your teenage years to protect your future health. Most important is to get enough calcium, especially since young women have the lowest intake of calcium of all age groups—less than 60 percent of the recommended amount of 1,200 mg daily. This is important, because by age seventeen, you've already built 91 percent of your bone mass, and most of the remaining percentage by your mid-twenties. After that, the goal is simply to maintain what you have achieved.

Your choice of foods can have an impact on the health of your bones (for information on the calcium content of many foods, see Appendix C). For each gram of protein consumed, 1 milligram of calcium is lost in urine. Protein increases the acid load of urine and requires calcium for use as a buffer. A diet high in sodium also causes calcium to be lost in the urine. For every gram of sodium you consume, urinary calcium increases by 26 milligrams. In short, the calcium used to keep your body balanced after eating fast foods and french fries comes at the expense of your bones.

Girls and young women also tend to skip breakfast more than any other meal. Studies have shown that not eating breakfast is associated with poor performance in school. Getting up a little early and getting your body going with yoga or exercise will stimulate your digestion and give you time for breakfast.

Menstruating Women

During your menstruating years, you can keep your menstrual cycle healthy with proper nutrition and eating habits. If you suffer from abdominal pains due to endometriosis, try cutting back on carbohydrates, such as rice, potatoes, pasta, corn, beets, and fruit juices. Add omega-9 fatty acids, such as olive, canola, and peanut oils. Eliminate foods with caffeine and tyramine (coffee, tea, colas, chocolate, aged cheeses, ale, sherry, and liquor). Adding omega-3 fatty acids may also help. You can take a supplement of omega-3 fatty acids or supplement your diet with flax seed oils or fish oils.

If you are struggling with PMS, stop using salt, sugar, alcohol, and caffeine for the week before your period, and limit your intake of fats. Add grains, fruits, and vegetables, and eat small meals often, even up to six per day. Studies have also shown that adding 1,200 mg of calcium supplements daily in the 2 weeks before your period can help reduce symptoms.

Pregnant Women

Conscious nutrition is particularly important when you are pregnant. However, this does not mean you need a lot of extra calories. In the first trimester, you do not need any extra calories, and in the second and third trimesters, you require only 300 calories per day more than your usual intake. But do make sure you consume enough vitamins and minerals, as this will have a major impact on the health of you and your baby. Take extra calcium, up to 1,200 milligrams daily, in addition to prenatal vitamins. Cottage cheese, milk, yogurt, and leafy green vegetables are excellent food sources of calcium. The most important vitamins and minerals are folic acid, iron, magnesium, zinc, and vitamins B_6, B_{12}, C, and E.

If you find you are unable to eat three large meals a day, try eating five smaller meals daily, and carry crackers, celery, or carrots with you to munch on if you feel hungry or queasy. If you are exercising regularly, be sure to eat enough to balance the extra calories you will burn off. Pregnancy is definitely not a time to lose weight. Avoid fasting, dieting, and skipping meals. Remember, you are eating for two. Try to avoid adding extra salt to your meals, especially if your hands and feet are swelling.

If you suffer from constipation, fresh carrot juice with a little spinach juice added can help you. Prune juice can also help. Be sure to drink plenty of water, at least eight glasses a day. For stubborn constipation, take six prunes and cover them with water. Leave them out overnight. In the morning, eat the prunes and drink the water.

Menopausal Women

Menopause is a time of life in which your choices will have a profound effect on your health. During perimenopause and menopause, your system is more sensitive. In addition to eating a lighter diet and timing your meals to match your activities, choose foods that are fresh and natural, as that will put less stress on the digestive system and liver.

BASIC ELEMENTS OF A HEALTHY DIET

- Eat lightly. Avoid overeating, undereating, and fad diets. Develop a healthy relationship with food.

- Digestion starts in the mouth. Chew your food well and eat mindfully. Your stomach does not have teeth!

- Eat only nutritious, sustaining, and healing foods that you can digest and eliminate within 24 hours. Avoid processed foods whenever possible.

- Choose vitamin, mineral, and herbal supplements that support each cycle of your life.

- Exercise and do yoga in the morning to stimulate your metabolism and stimulate your digestive system.

- Give your digestive system a rest by eating lightly one day each week. Whatever you eat you have to digest. One-third to one-half of your body's energy goes toward digesting your food.

- Take your meals early in the day and at midday, when your digestive energy is at its height. Avoid eating at night.

- At 4:00 P.M. each day, eat a banana and some raisins. Try eating a banana with mango powder and lemon for potassium balance. Potassium is very important to a woman's health and will help regulate your biorhythm.

- Monitor your elimination and transit time. The more efficiently you digest and absorb your food, the healthier you will be.

- Relax after each meal.

Cleansing

For most of us it is hard to maintain a balanced diet. As a result of busy schedules, travel, exposure to pollution, and stress, you may eat more processed food, junk food, or heavy food than you can healthfully tolerate. As a result, you may begin to feel lethargic, lose your appetite, or experience chronic indigestion. The continuous buildup and presence of toxins from eating an imbalanced diet can eventually lead to many health problems.

If your diet is seriously out of balance, see a nutrition counselor or a cleansing health practitioner, or attempt to eliminate the hard-to-digest foods from your diet. Your digestive system is especially sensitive. Starvation diets are not considered to be cleansing; they can be shocking and harmful to your body. If you want to experience the effects of a deep cleansing of your digestive system, there are many qualified health practitioners who can help you. Cleansing your body and eliminating toxins can trigger the release of negative emotional patterns and help you to confront your food addictions. The support of a professional can be vital for the successful completion of a cleansing program. Cleansing programs can give you the time and space you need to develop healthier dietary habits.

There are certain individuals who cannot tolerate hunger, and it is recommended that, even on a cleansing diet, they eat every few hours. Listen to your body's messages as you cleanse. Food can be used as medicine to heal you, and the results can be amazing! Your kitchen can be your nearest pharmacy.

Yoga Set to Support Digestion

This particular yoga set works as a tune-up for your digestive system, as do the exercises in Chapter 2.

Breath for Elimination

To benefit your digestive system, do this kriya regularly (not missing even one day), but no more than twice daily on an empty stomach. Sit in Easy Pose, with your hands on your knees. Make a round bead of your mouth and drink in as much air as you can into your stomach in short, continuous "sips" like short inhalations. When you can't sip/inhale any more, close your mouth and hold your breath in as you roll your stomach left and right as long as possible. Keep the Neck Lock applied (holding the chin steady and pulled in toward the spine). Churn the stomach area, pulling the navel area back and around, left and right. When you can no longer hold the breath in, slowly and gently (not powerfully) exhale through the nose in one continuous stream. Repeat the exercise twice—a total of three rounds of inhaling and exhaling. Relax.

Digestive Massage

Sitting on your heels in Baby Pose, bring your forehead to the floor in front of you. Relax your arms at your sides with your palms facing upward near your feet (Baby Pose). From the waistline, slowly move your hips to the left and right. Imagine you are wagging a heavy tail attached to your tailbone. Continue moving your hips from side to side for 2–3 minutes (beginners start with 1–3 minutes). To release the posture, stop moving the hips and bring your palms to the floor at the sides of your head. Press the palms as you lift up to a sitting position. Then lie down and relax for 5 minutes.

Benefits Baby Pose is a relaxed posture that brings circulation to the heart, eyes, and head. It helps to cleanse the upper lungs and can help you relax when you are anxious or tense. Moving the hips side to side in this posture is wonderful for massaging the internal digestive organs and will assist in the elimination of waste from the body.

Leg Lifts for Digestion

Lie on your back. Relax your arms by the side of your body, or place the hands under the buttocks/lower back to support your back. Point your toes forward and lift your legs 3 feet off the ground. Hold the posture with Long, Deep Breathing. Keep up for 2 minutes. If you need a break, relax your legs down and resume the posture as soon as you can.

Benefits This posture works on the gall bladder and slims the waistline. The angle of 3 feet is important to get the full benefit of this exercise.

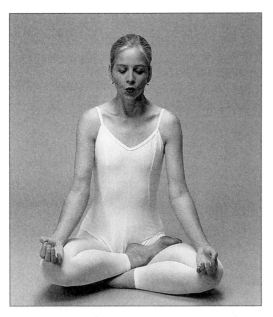

Breath for Elimination

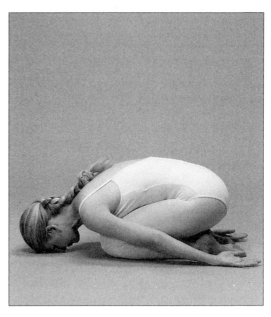

Digestive Massage

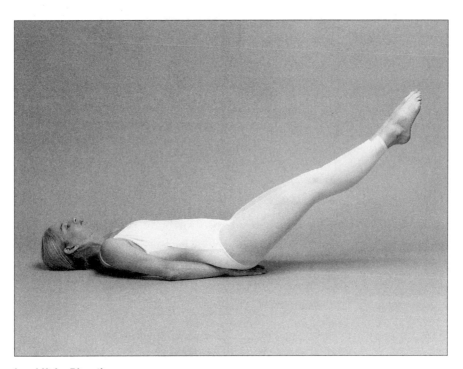

Leg Lift for Digestion

Rolling on the Spine

Lie on your back. Lift your legs up and stretch them so you can grab your toes with your hands. Roll back and forth from the base of your spine to the top of your spine. Keep holding your toes and rolling. Do your best! If you cannot grab the toes, hold your legs behind your knees. Keep working toward doing the exercise. Continue for 3 minutes (beginners start with 1–3 minutes).

Benefits This exercise benefits your circulation by helping to open the capillaries. It also strengthens the nervous system. During menopause, these kinds of strenuous exercises are excellent. There is a saying in Kundalini Yoga: "Keep up and you'll be kept up!"

Alternate Nostril Breathing

Immediately sit in Easy Pose. Cover the right nostril with your left thumb and inhale through the left nostril. Use your little finger of the left hand to close the left nostril as you exhale through the right. Continue to inhale left and exhale right. Remember to coordinate the mantra *Sat Naam* with the breathing for focusing and synchronizing mind and body. Continue for 3 minutes.

Benefits This exercise helps calm the nervous system. It is also an excellent meditation by itself for balancing the body and mind during menopause.

Bear Grip Mudra

Sit in Easy Pose. Raise both hands up a few inches in front of your chest, elbows parallel to the floor. Form Bear Grip Mudra as follows: Face your left palm out and away from you, your right palm toward the left, and curl the fingers of both hands so they hook each other. Lock the thumbs of each hand over the little fingers of the opposite hand. Holding this posture with your right arm, inhale as the chin goes over to your left shoulder, and exhale as it turns to the right. Continue for 1–3 minutes.

Benefits This simple exercise helps to create healthy thyroid and parathyroid glands, which are often referred to as the guardians of health and beauty.

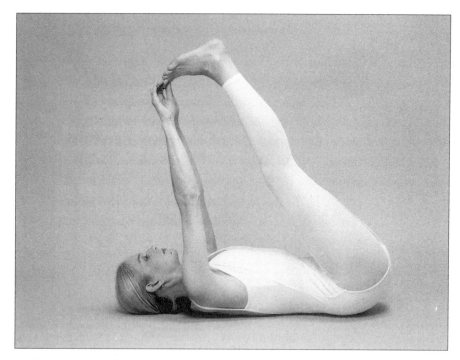

Rolling on the Spine

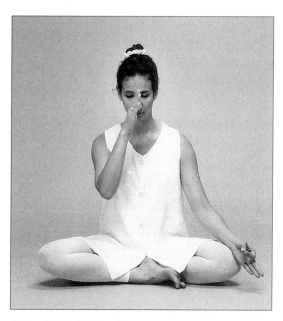

Alternate Nostril Breathing

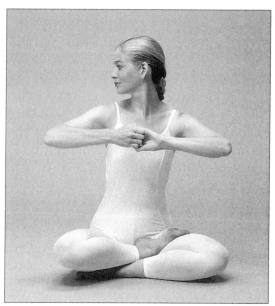

Bear Grip Mudra

During menopause, Bear Grip Mudra can help women stabilize the fluctuations they may experience in the functioning of these glands.

Arm Circles

Sitting in Easy Pose, stretch your arms out to the side, keeping them parallel to the floor. Swing them backward in a circular motion, as if swimming backward. Make big circles and continue for 1 minute while doing Breath of Fire. Then inhale and hold the breath, bringing your hands to your shoulders (right hand on right shoulder, left hand on left shoulder). While you hold your breath, mentally circulate the energy to all the cells in your body. Exhale and relax, letting the body experience the flow of energy.

Benefits This exercise helps to balance your electromagnetic field and stabilize your outer projection.

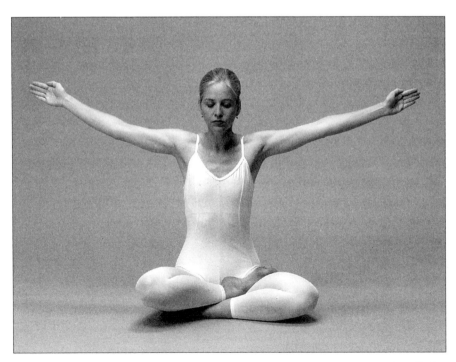

Arm Circles

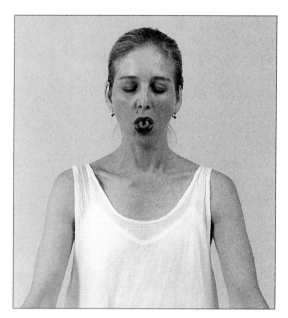

Sitali Pranayam

Sitali Pranayam

Sit in a comfortable position. Stick your tongue out of your mouth, just beyond your lips, and curl up the sides of your tongue into a "U." Inhale deeply through your rolled tongue, and exhale through your nose. Continue this breath pattern for a minimum of 2–3 minutes.

Benefits This is a powerful healing technique for many illnesses, including fever and digestive disorders. At first your tongue may taste bitter, and then it will become sweet. You can also practice this breath technique twenty-six times in the morning and twenty-six times at night to enjoy its healing effects.

Recipes for Health and Healing

Ms. Whiz—A Breakfast Drink for Women

You can use this recipe to take your daily dose of sesame or almond oil. If you are watching your weight, you might consider using 2 tablespoons of protein powder in place of the cold-pressed oil.

1 ripe banana

8 oz. orange juice

1 tbsp. liquid chlorophyll

2 tsp. rice bran syrup (for mineral balance)

2 tsp. cold-pressed almond oil or sesame oil

Blend until frothy.

Mung Beans and Rice

Mung beans and rice cooked in this fashion are considered a *predigested food.* That is, the foods are very easy to digest, and the protein and nutrients in them are easy to absorb. This particular recipe is based on Yogi Bhajan's recipe for a traditional dish called kitcheree. This dish has everything you need; you can use this as a new and healthy comfort food.

1 cup mung beans

1 cup basmati rice

9 cups water

4–6 cups assorted vegetables (carrots, celery, zucchini, broccoli, Swiss chard, etc.), chopped

1/2 cup oil (olive oil or any pure vegetable oil)

2 onions, chopped

8–10 cloves garlic, minced

1/3 cup ginger root, minced

1 heaping tsp. turmeric

1/2 tsp. pepper

1 heaping tsp. garam masala

1 tsp. red chilies, crushed

2 bay leaves

Seeds of 5 cardamom pods

1 tbsp. sweet basil, chopped

Salt or soy sauce to taste

Soak beans for at least 8 hours (or precook for 30 minutes). Rinse beans and rice. Bring water to a boil; add rice and beans, and simmer over medium heat. Prepare vegetables and add to rice and beans. Heat oil in a large frying pan; add onions, garlic, and ginger, and sauté over medium heat until brown. Add spices (not basil or salt). When nicely done, combine sautéed onion mixture with rice and beans. Stir often to prevent rice and beans from scorching. Add herbs, and continue to cook over medium-low heat, stirring often, until done. The consistency should be rich, thick, and souplike, with ingredients barely discernible. Season with salt or soy sauce. Note: Eliminate or reduce spices to taste.

Serves 4–6.

Mango Lassi—A Refreshing Yogurt Drink

This cooling drink is high in calcium and protein. The mangoes are also considered excellent for sexual health.

2 medium mangoes (very ripe)	6 ice cubes
2 cups fresh plain yogurt	8 tsp. rose water
2 tbsp. maple syrup or honey	

Peel and slice mangoes. Combine all ingredients in a blender at high speed. Serves 4–6.

Ginger Tea

This tea is an excellent tonic for women, as is ginger in general (include generous amounts in your cooking). Taken during your menstrual period, Ginger Tea can help keep you energized and soothe your digestion. This tea can also help relieve the aches and discomfort of fever and help soothe the nervous system.

Boil 4 or 5 slices of fresh ginger root in 3 cups of water. Add honey and milk to taste, if desired.

Energy Tea

A boiled infusion of basil and turmeric, strained to make a tea and taken as 1 cup four times daily, will keep you steady and give you energy. Also take 1 oz. of lemon juice and a ¼ oz. of ginger juice (made with a juicer or obtained at a juice bar) mixed together. Sip slowly or add water to make a drink.

Drink to Balance Minerals in Your Body

6 prunes	3 bananas
6 figs	8 oz. plain yogurt
1 handful raisins	

Soak prunes, figs, and raisins overnight in water (enough to cover the fruit). In the morning, add the bananas and yogurt. Blend together with ice and the water in which the dried fruit was soaked. Divide this mixture into three equal parts and drink throughout the day.

If you suffer from cold hands and feet, add 10–15 soaked saffron threads to the drink. You can also make this filling, nutritious drink a complete meal by adding a handful of nuts before blending. (Don't use it to replace a meal for more than one day and be sure that you have a hearty meal of steamed vegetables the next day.)

"Yogi Mush" for Clear Skin

Your skin is your largest organ. One of its functions is to eliminate toxins from the body (as you sweat). If you eat this dish regularly, it will help you keep your skin beautiful and cleanse your intestines. It is a low-calorie, high-vitamin and -mineral dish that can also help you lose weight.

4 celery stalks	1 sprig mint
1 bunch parsley	$\frac{1}{2}$ tsp. ground black pepper
4–5 medium zucchini	1 cup cottage cheese

Steam celery, parsley, zucchini, and mint for about 15 minutes until soft. Puree with black pepper. Serve with cottage cheese.

Makes about 2 servings.

"Colon Cleanser"

This recipe stimulates and balances the metabolism and works on the thyroid, pituitary, and pineal glands.

12 almonds (without skins)
6 prunes, pitted

Soak both the almonds and the pitted prunes overnight in 8 ounces of water. In the morning, blend them together until liquified as completely as possible. Drink as a morning drink. After the almonds soak in the water for 6 hours they begin to sprout, creating nitrogen. This nitrogen and the almonds, even more potent when blended with the iron in the prunes, act as a colon cleanser and a metabolism stimulant.

Sesame Yogurt Dressing

When eating raw vegetables, add a healthy dressing to assist in digestion. The following recipe is a balanced, delicious dressing that is especially good during pregnancy for preventing the gas that may result from eating raw vegetables.

4 sprigs parsley	2 tbsp. lemon juice
1 stalk celery, chopped	1/2 tsp. salt
1/2 cup sesame seeds	1/4 tsp. ground black pepper
1/4 small onion, chopped	1 tsp. honey
1 clove garlic, sliced	2 tbsp. soy sauce
1/2 cup raw sesame oil	1 cup plain yogurt
1 tbsp. vinegar	

Blend all ingredients until smooth and serve.
Makes 3 cups.

Yogi Bhajan's "Yogi Tea"

The basic tea tonic in our yoga community—healing and delicious!

3 whole cloves	10 oz. water
4 green cardamom pods	1/4 tsp. black tea
1/2 stick cinnamon	1/2 cup milk
1 ginger root, sliced	Honey to taste
1/4 tsp. ground black pepper	

Boil spices in water for 10–15 minutes. Add black tea and steep for 2 minutes. Add milk, then reheat to the boiling point. Remove immediately from the stove and strain. Add honey to taste.

To make 2 quarts, use 20 cardamom pods, 20 peppercorns, 15 cloves, 3 cinnamon sticks, and 1 tbsp. black tea. Boil at least 30 minutes. Add 1 quart milk and proceed as previously directed. Make a new batch each time so that your tea is fresh and balanced.

Yogi Tea is a staple of the yogi's diet. This balanced blend of herbs stimulates digestion and elimination. The scent of simmering yogi tea stimulates all of your senses and the taste is fantastic.

For liver health and additional cleansing, place a covered cup of raw yogi tea (without milk or honey) on your bedside table. Drink the tea after you wake up and before you get out of bed.

GARLIC, ONIONS, AND GINGER

Considered the "trinity roots," garlic, onions, and ginger are the basis of most of the healing recipes in the science of Ayurveda. These roots are supportive of the health of your tissues and immune system. They support your endocrine glands, help reduce blood pressure (garlic is used to help reduce cholesterol), and increase circulatory health. Include these roots in your diet to promote health and healing.

Gut Reaction

Emotions and the intestinal tract are closely connected; stress and digestion are linked, as are stress and intestinal diseases. We are all aware of the way physical sensations of the intestinal tract are associated with fear. When you feel fear, signals transmitted through the brain to the hypothalamus and brain stem alter blood flow to the abdomen and may cause nausea or loss of bowel control. Although it may be a less potent stimulus, the stress of daily life can have an adverse effect on the intestinal tract. Yoga can play an important role in combating digestive reactions to these everyday stresses and emotions. Yoga stimulates the parasympathetic nervous system and activates the nerves that help us relax and control the intestinal tract, thereby aiding the digestive process and enhancing our peace of mind.

Short and Gentle Yoga Session for Improving Digestion

1. Tune in.

2. Breath of Fire for 3–5 minutes to stimulate digestive fire, strengthen your nervous system, and help you break addictive habits.

3. Spinal Flex and Spinal Twist to warm up.

4. Forward Bend performed gently without collapsing your spine.

5. Sat Kriya for 3–7 minutes to stimulate your energy. You can do Sat Kriya while sitting in a chair if Rock Pose (sitting on your heels) is too challenging for you.

6. Relax.

7. Sitali Pranayam.

Longer Yoga Session for Improving Digestion

1. Tune in.

2. Breath of Fire for 3 minutes to stimulate digestive fire, strengthen your nervous system, and help you break addictive habits.

3. Spinal Flex and Spinal Twist to warm up.

4. Yoga Set to Support Digestion and Elimination.

5. Relax.

6. Sitali Pranayam.

QUESTIONS FOR FURTHER GROWTH

- Keep a journal of what you eat for 3 days. Assess your diet. Do you eat five servings of fruits and vegetables daily? If not, can you either substitute fruits and vegetables for less healthy foods or add your favorites to your diet?

- Do you secretly suffer from food addictions or a constant fear of gaining weight? If so, make an appointment to see your doctor or health-care practitioner to help you conquer these challenges.

- Do you eat and snack right before bed? If so, can you adjust your snacks or your dinner to avoid eating too much before bed for healthier digestion?

- What stage of life are you in? Follow the recommendations for increased nutrition for the stage of life you are in now.

- Choose three healthy habits to incorporate into your diet lifestyle. Which ones did you choose and why?

CHAPTER

10 Self-Healing

The process of self-healing is the privilege of every being. Self-healing is not a miracle, nor is self-healing a dramatization of the personality, as though you could do something superior. Self-healing is a genuine process of the relationship between the physical body and the infinite power of the soul.

—Yogi Bhajan

ealing means to "make whole." When the yogis speak of healing, they mean something other than curing, which refers to *eliminating* a disease or illness. A person who is "healed" may also have a disease or illness. The yogis view the physical body as more than the sum of its parts, and as such you can still be whole and complete, even if a part of you is not fully functioning. When your body is in rhythm with the infinite consciousness, there is health, or "ease." When this rhythm is lost, there is *dis*-ease. Notes Yogi Bhajan: "Disease is nothing but an out-of-rhythm body . . . or mind." The process of self-healing allows you to feel liberated and whole throughout your life, even as you encounter times of both conventional health and illness.

Using the proper tools, you have the ability to profoundly influence your own physical, mental, and spiritual states. This natural human facility for self-healing is the essence of yoga. The effects from the practice of Kundalini Yoga are lasting and can have a permanent impact on the quality of your life. If you approach your personal growth from the perspective of empowered ability and if you believe in your capacity to create positive change, you can experience self-healing.

Whatever your temporary circumstances, you can live in the timeless reality of your soul. If you feel gripped by stress, confused by the polarities of your preferences and desires, and disturbed by the ups and downs of life, the yogis would say you are in a dream, forgetting your natural state—the constant experience of the divine within you, your true identity—*Sat Naam.*

Living in the awareness of the divine does not mean that yogis do not experience emotion, pain, and pleasure. They certainly do. But a true yogini does not get attached to any particular emotion and can process each emotion or sensation as it comes. By not limiting yourself to a narrow range of feelings or reactions, the whole array of feelings and emotions are there for you to experience. Experiencing the full range of your sensations, you are truly present to the rhythm of life. Self-healing is the ability to care for your body, process your emotions and feelings in a healthy way, and direct your mind to match your inner truth so you can experience the full rhythm of life. The practice of self-healing can, indeed, cure disease and help you transcend a diseased state if it persists.

Throughout your life, you will face many unexpected challenges. The meditations and exercises here are representative of a vast technology of self-healing in the science of Kundalini Yoga. To get the most benefit from any one meditation or exercise, practice it each day for 40 days. This period is needed to break the pattern of the old negative habits and to help solidify the positive pattern you are creating.

The Reality of Illness, Trauma, and Disease

Keytiaa dookh bhook sad maar
Eh bhe data teree daataar.
(Many are those who endure distress, privation, and constant abuse.
Even these are Your Gifts, O Great Giver.)
—GURU NANAK-JAAPJI

The experience of living in the human body is filled with challenges on every level. Living in the world requires balancing the polarities of health and illness, pain and pleasure, which determine our temporal experience. When you attain a yogic perspective on the polarities of life, you can move through them without being affected by them. But how is this possible? How can anyone not prefer pleasure to pain or health to illness?

Yogis believe that this earth plane is a school, a classroom for your soul. The lessons of both health and illness, of pleasure and pain, are equally important aspects of the learning process. Some yogic teachings explain that this world of polarities is actually designed to disillusion us so that we will search for something more. We are directed through the experience of pain and challenge as well as the distraction of pleasure and health to strive to understand something that is beyond this earthly plane. Suffering the usual "slings and arrows" of life is intended to move us toward the discovery of our own Divine Self as well as the Universal Consciousness that connects us all.

Illness, disease, and trauma come to many who live healthy lives, have healthy habits, and do good deeds. Long lives can also come to those who have unhealthy habits! We hear about the suffering of young people facing cancer, early deaths that we cannot easily understand. Women especially may have to cope with the deeper wounds of losing children to war, illness, accidents, and so on.

The effects of trauma are often insidious. A woman's trauma from sexual, physical, and psychological abuse deeply affects both her subtle and physical bodies. As a human being, you have the right to live with respect and love. Do not put up with any abuses that can be prevented. At times, life itself may seem to abuse us. Accidents happen, and we may see things we wish we never had. Violence and abuse can create a pattern of guilt and shame. These can then lead to self-abuse, which you carry with you in your thinking or actions. If you are dealing with trauma, the path of yoga can be empowering and healing. In addition to working with the meditations and exercises in this book, you can consult a teacher or therapist who can allow you the time and space to resolve old feelings of hurt and to promote new feelings of self-worth and self-acceptance.

As a yogini, be willing to encounter the process of life instead of resisting the changes and challenges that will beset you. Practice accepting both the value of your life and the reality of your death. By developing the yogic attitude toward life experience, you will remain balanced in both mind and body and will be able serve those you love in all situations. You will become fearless in the face of all that life can deliver and will remain graceful through all challenges. It is worth repeating the words of Yogi Bhajan: "It's not the life that you live—it's the courage that you bring to it."

DR.'S NOTES

Fall seven times, stand up eight.

—Japanese proverb

The body has an enormous capacity to heal itself. The breathing, meditations, and poses presented in this book help the body help itself: Breathing helps to bring oxygen to the distant reaches of the body, meditations help to oppose the negative effects of stress, and the poses keep us strong and flexible. But much self healing can be accomplished by avoiding self-destructive behaviors. Not smoking helps each breath to better oxygenate the body and reduces our risks of heart disease and cancer. Exercising strengthens our heart and burns excess calories. Eating well and in moderation reduces the risk of obesity, a major contributor to many diseases as well as to lowered self-esteem. Chewing our food well is a great aid to digestion. And practicing yoga and other types of meditative practices helps to relieve stress. The composite of these preventive health measures keeps the natural healing powers of our bodies performing at their best and lowers the chances that external forms of healing will be needed. In addition, taking care of mind and body helps us build the courage needed to get up each time we are knocked down.

Self-Healing Meditations for Body, Mind, and Spirit

Self-healing takes place on several levels. You can practice healing yourself on the physical level with the exercises and postures that work directly on your body systems. Self-healing also occurs on the mental level. Meditation is a powerful tool for mastering the level of the mind so you can cut through the self-destructive thoughts that lead to self-destructive behaviors. Yogi Bhajan teaches that because a woman has the ability to access both hemispheres of her brain, she can become her own "psychiatrist." Through meditation, self-affirming thinking, and development of a positive approach to life, you can learn to solve your own problems and heal yourself. You can also experience healing on the spiritual level. *Spirit* has come to have different meanings for many people. If you have difficulty connecting with your "spirit," consider defining the spiritual dimension as that which represents you in relation to the entire cosmos. This includes your feeling of connection with your family, friends, and community, and your relationship to the natural world. The spiritual dimension can also include the level of acceptance and contentment you bring to your daily life.

The Kriya meditations and breathing exercises that follow can lead you into the yogic experience of self-healing on the levels of body, mind, and spirit. Take your time to experience them. Choose one that addresses a particular need you have, and practice it for at least 40 days. Keep a journal and monitor your progress.

Meditation for Emotional Balance— From Insecurity to Freedom

Before you begin this meditation, drink a full 8-ounce glass of water. Sit in Easy Pose (cross-legged) or in a comfortable seated posture, and place your arms across your chest. Lock your hands under your armpits. Keep your palms open and against your body, as if you were hugging yourself. Raise your

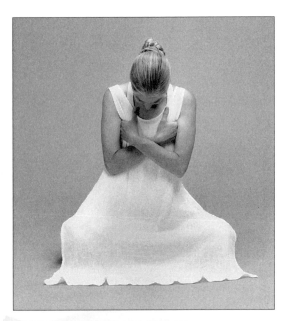

Meditation for Emotional Balance

shoulders tight up toward your earlobes. Apply the Neck Lock, bringing your chin down and in toward your spine. Close your eyes. Hold this posture and let your breath find its own rhythm. Your breath will automatically slow. Continue meditating like this for 3 minutes. You can gradually increase the time of this meditation to 11 minutes.

Benefits Do this meditation whenever you are highly emotional, upset, or worried. If you are in a tense situation and feel out of control, it is important at that time to pay special attention to your water balance and breath rate. Both dehydration and overdrinking will add to your worries and upset. (Most women do not overdrink water, but it is possible: 6–8 glasses of pure water daily is a healthy amount to prevent dehydration.) In this meditation, drinking water and pulling your shoulders up to your ears (locking your upper body) will break the pattern of upset and negative emotion and enable you to return to a relaxed state.

Meditation for Regulating Eating Habits

Sit in Easy Pose. Breathe long and deeply through your left nostril only, blocking your right nostril with your right thumb. After you inhale completely, suspend the breath in the body for a comfortable length of time. Exhale and hold the breath out as well. Continue in a balanced way without straining. Meditate in this way for 31 minutes. It generally takes 90 days to experience the full effects of this meditation.

Benefits This meditation balances the hemispheres of your brain, which allows you to have an impact on your own habits.

Ten-Step Meditation to Peace

This meditation erases bad memories and helps you to transcend painful experiences.

1. Lower your eyelids until your eyes are only one-tenth open. Concentrate on the tip of your nose. Silently repeat the mantra *Wha Hay Guroo* (pronounced *wah-hey-goo-roo*), the mantra of ecstasy and timeless wisdom, in the following sequence:

   Wha—Mentally focus on your right eye.
   Hay—Mentally focus on your left eye.
   Guroo—Mentally focus on the tip of your nose.

2. Inhale and recall the encounter, incident, or experience you want to erase.

3. Exhale and mentally repeat *Wha Hay Guroo* again, using the above mental focus.

4. Inhale and suspend your breath as you mentally relive the feelings of the experience.

5. Exhale, hold your breath out, and repeat the mantra again, using the mental focus.

6. Inhale and suspend your breath. Reverse roles in the encounter you are remembering. Become the other person and relive the experience from his or her perspective.

7. Exhale and hold your breath out. Repeat the mantra again, using the mental focus.

8. Inhale and suspend the breath. Forgive the other person and forgive yourself.

9. Exhale and mentally repeat the mantra.

10. Inhale. Let go of the incident and release it to the universe.

Says Yogi Bhajan: "This meditation takes care of phobias, fears, and neuroses. It can remove unsettling thoughts from the past that surface in the present. It can take difficult situations in the present and release them into the hands of infinity." Practicing this meditation can train you to develop a pattern of processing and releasing your disturbing thoughts and experiences, instead of dwelling on negativity.

Nine-Minute Meditation to Alleviate Stress

Stress is detrimental to your health and causes hyperactivity of your adrenal glands. These spikes of adrenaline are designed to quickly supply oxygen and energy in an emergency situation, but over a longer period of time, excess adrenaline can lead to problems such as ulcers, high blood pressure, and loss of appetite. Constant stress can also lead to headaches, depression, chronic fatigue syndrome, adult-onset diabetes, and digestive ailments. Stress can upset your immune system, lower your resistance to disease, and reduce your memory.

Meditation and relaxation have a powerful effect on reducing the intensity and impact of stress on your body and mind. Practicing meditations like the one that follows can help you to conquer the daily stresses of modern life. Although this meditation takes only 9 minutes, *it can make a huge difference*

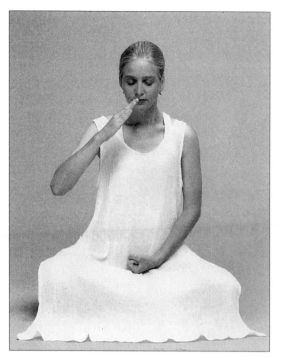
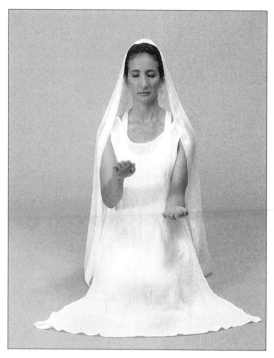

Nine-Minute Meditation to Alleviate Stress (1)   **Nine-Minute Meditation to Alleviate Stress (2)**

in your life. Remember to breathe and focus on the mantra *Sat* on your inhalation, and on *Naam* on your exhalation throughout the meditation.

1. Sitting in Easy Pose or in a chair, bend your right elbow so your forearm is in front of your body and parallel to the floor. Your wrist and fingers are straight, and the palm of your hand is facing downward. Keep your eyes closed and focused on the center of your chin. Without bending your wrist, move your forearm up and down quickly, like a fan, from the tip of your nose to your navel point. Put all your energy into the movement. After 1 minute, make a fist with your left hand as you continue the motion with your right hand for 2 more minutes.

Benefits This fanning motion relaxes your heart.

2. Still seated, place your arms by your side and bend your elbows, raising your forearms so that they are parallel to the floor. Your hands should be pointing forward, your left palm facing downward (toward

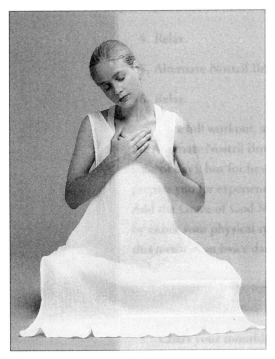

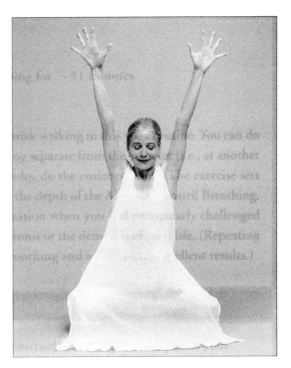

Nine-Minute Meditation to Alleviate Stress (3)　　**Nine-Minute Meditation** to Alleviate Stress (4)

earth) and your right palm facing upward (toward the heavens). Alternately move each forearm up and down 6–8 inches from the parallel, as if you were bouncing balls with your hands. Continue this motion for 3 minutes.

Benefits This part of the meditation restores balance to the qualities of earth and heaven within you, creating a deep relaxation in the body and mind.

3. Remain seated and place your hands on the center of your chest (the heart center) with your right hand over your left. Close your eyes. Begin stretching and bending your neck, bringing your left ear toward your left shoulder and your right ear toward your right shoulder. Continue this motion without stress, in a rhythmic manner. Relax into the motion for 2 minutes.

Benefits This exercise helps to adjust your neck and release tension from your shoulders, neck, and face.

4. Stretch your arms over your head with arms straight and your fingers extended up and open as widely as possible. Squeeze all the muscles in your body as you continue to stretch upward and breathe. Stretch like this for 1 minute, then relax.

Benefits Completing the meditation this way integrates new patterns of relaxation into your body and releases any remaining tension. Remember to relax after you complete the entire meditation.

Meditation to Create Self-Love

When you are fearful and self-critical, your nervous system is negatively affected. "Love doesn't rule you," says Yogi Bhajan. "What rules you is fear, phenomenal fear. Through this kriya, love can be invoked and fear can be reduced." This meditation not only helps conquer fear but also stimulates your energy, opens your heart chakra (the center of love and compassion), and gives you strength.

1. Sit in a comfortable posture with your spine straight. Place your right hand palm down a maximum of 6 inches over the crown of your head. Bend your left elbow in by your side and bring your left palm up to shoulder height with the palm facing forward. Focus your closed eyes downward toward your chin. Breathe Long, Deep Breaths with a feeling of self-affection. Bless yourself and bless the world. Try to breathe only one breath per minute: inhale for 20 seconds, hold 20 seconds, exhale for 20 seconds. (Work up to this One-Minute Breath by beginning with 5 seconds for the inhalation, 5 seconds holding, and 5 seconds for the exhalation.) Hold the posture and slow breathing for 5–11 minutes. Then slowly move into the next posture.

2. Still seated, extend your arms straight out from your shoulders, parallel to the ground and palms facing down toward the ground. Stretch out from your shoulders and armpits. Keep the same eye focus on your chin and breathe Long, Deep Breaths. Hold this posture for 1–3 minutes, and then move slowly to the next posture.

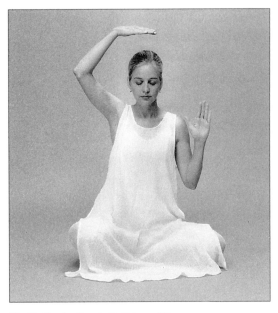

Meditation to Create Self-Love (1)

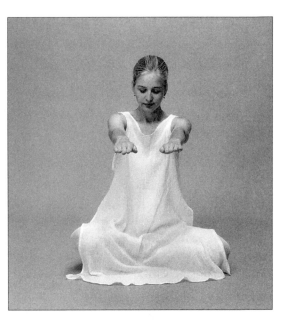

Meditation to Create Self-Love (2)

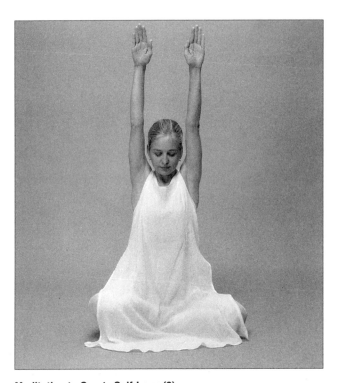

Meditation to Create Self-Love (3)

3. Stretch your arms straight up in the air, with no bend in the elbows. Keep your eyes focused on your chin and continue Long, Deep Breathing. Hold this posture for 1–3 minutes. To end this meditation, inhale deeply and hold your breath for 10 seconds while you consciously stretch, as if you were pulling yourself off the floor. Tighten all the muscles in your body! Exhale. Repeat this ending sequence two more times, then relax.

Meditation for a Woman's Arc Lines

Remember that a woman has two arc lines, one from ear to ear over the head (similar to a halo) and the second forming an arc from nipple to nipple across her chest, the heart center chakra (see Chapter 1). This heart chakra arc line reflects a woman's life experiences. The following meditation helps strengthen your heart chakra arc line and release negative impressions so you can be radiant and compassionate.

1. Sit in Easy Pose or in another comfortable posture. Make your hands into fists and extend the first two fingers straight out. Keep these two extended fingers touching, held side by side, remaining straight. The ring and pinkie fingers will be held down in the middle of the palm, with the thumb.

2. With your arms down at your sides, bend your elbows, bringing your hands in front of each shoulder, palms facing forward. The two extended fingers point straight up. Focus your eyes on the tip of your nose.

3. Movement: Swing your hands from Arc Line A to Arc Line B in a continuous sweeping motion. Regulate your cross movement so that there are no breaks in the movement.

4. Bring the two hands together in front of the chest, touching only the extended fingertips of the right hand with the extended fingers of the left hand. The palms will be facing each other but not touching.

5. Swing the hands out to the sides, palms facing forward, with a space of about 24 inches between the hands. The extended fingers of the

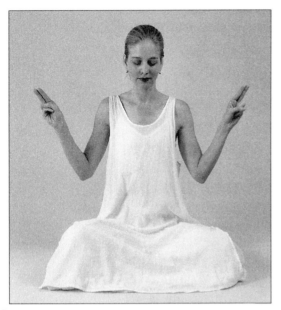

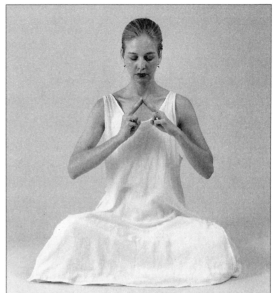

Arc Line A

Arc Line B

right hand will be at a 45-degree angle out to the right; the extended fingers of the left hand will be at a 45-degree angle out to the left.

6. Chant the mantra *Har* (striking the "r" on the roof of your mouth). This mantra can be translated to mean "Infinity" or "Infinite Creator." Continue moving the hands in a rhythmic pattern at a steady pace as if you were drumming, chanting the mantra with the movement. Continue for 3–14 mintues.

7. Relax.

Breath of Fire for Radiance and Victory

Practice this coordinated posture and breathing exercise daily to improve your quality of radiance, brighten and strengthen your aura, and increase your ability to conquer stress. It is your radiance that causes your presence to have an impact. When your presence has an impact on those around you, you can move forward with commitment, strength, and success.

Sit in Easy Pose, in another comfortable posture, or in a chair. Stretch your arms over your head, extended to a 60-degree angle, creating a Y. Curl your hands into a fist, leaving your thumbs out and pointing up. Face your hands forward. Hold this posture as you begin Breath of Fire for 1–3 minutes. To end, inhale and suspend your breath. Open and close your fists very quickly, alternating your thumb inside and outside of your closed fist for 15 seconds. Then stretch your hands up and meet your thumbs over the crown of your head. Exhale as you relax your hands down in an arclike motion around your body. Relax and experience the positive effects of this exercise.

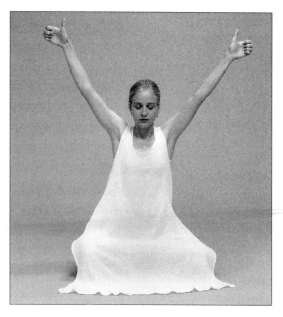

Breath of Fire

You can also practice Breath of Fire in Easy Pose while holding your hands in Gyan Mudra (thumb and index finger forming a circle) on your knees. You can slowly build up this practice to 31 minutes. Another good sequence for learning Breath of Fire is to alternate Breath of Fire with Long, Deep Breathing. Try doing a minute of Breath of Fire followed by a minute of Long, Deep Breathing. You can then increase the practice to 3 minutes of Breath of Fire and 3 minutes of Long, Deep Breathing.

Benefits Breath of Fire stimulates your parasympathetic nervous system and cuts through stress to restore you to a balanced state of mind, body, and soul. Breath of Fire also stimulates the fire element in you and strengthens your ability to digest and transform food into fuel to energize your system. If your fire element is out of balance, you lose your power and presence. Practicing Breath of Fire will give you confidence and a strong sense of self-esteem.

Breath to Relax the Mind and Calm Strong Desires and Attachments

Form your mouth into the shape of an O. Inhale a Long, Deep Breath through the O of your mouth. Exhale through your nose. Continue until you feel the effects. Whenever you are breathing through your mouth, make sure you are using diaphragmatic breathing. If you feel dizzy, stop the practice, take a few breaths, and start again.

Breath to Transform Anger

Use this breath to release anger appropriately and quickly. Form your tongue into a U shape and stick it out just beyond your lips. Inhale Long, Deep Breaths through your mouth, through the curl of your tongue. Exhale deeply through your nose. This is called Sitali Pranayam (pictured on page 200). It can help you cool down when you are hot, have a fever, or have digestive difficulties. This breath is very relaxing. If you practice it twenty-six times each morning and evening, you will experience many benefits. You can also use this technique to help you resist food cravings. Curl your tongue as previously described, but extend your tongue a little bit more. Inhale through your mouth and exhale through your mouth while keeping your tongue curled.

The One-Minute Breath for Transforming Depression into Divinity

The One-Minute Breath is an extraordinary yogic practice. It can quickly adjust your mental and emotional states and calm your body systems. To practice the One-Minute Breath, inhale slowly for 20 seconds, suspend the breath in your body for 20 seconds, and exhale slowly for 20 seconds, then repeat the sequence. It may take time to work up to 20 seconds. Start with a time that is comfortable for you (5 to 10 seconds). You will benefit from the practice even at these beginning stages. Practice the sequence at that stage for up to 11 minutes. Add a few seconds when you can, without straining, until you reach the 20 seconds. The One-Minute Breath will help you to handle all the stresses we experience living in our modern fast-paced society. A woman can also do the One-Minute Breath prior to intercourse if she is trying to conceive.

Meditation for Intuition and Conquering Fear

Sit in Easy Pose (cross-legged) or in a chair. Relax your elbows by your side and bring your forearms parallel to the floor and angled out so that they follow the angle of your legs if you are in the cross-legged posture. With your palms facing upward, bring the fingertips of each together. This is called Closed Lotus Mudra. Close your eyes and focus them on your brow point. Hold this eye focus. Inhale deeply and exhale. Hold your breath out and mentally repeat the mantra sequence *Saa Taa Naa Maa* four times. You will hold your breath out for a total of sixteen counts. Inhale deeply, exhale, and begin the sequence again. Continue this sequence with the mental chanting at your brow for 11 minutes. To end the meditation, inhale, hold your breath briefly, then relax.

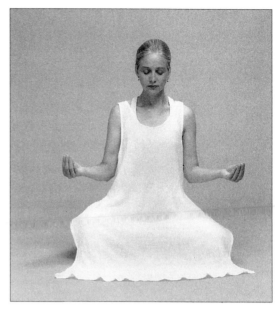

Meditation for Intuition and Conquering Fear

Benefits As you hold your breath out, you automatically trigger the release of chronic fears, including the fear of death. As you provoke and release fears physiologically and mentally with the breath pattern, your eye focus and mental vibration stimulate your pituitary gland and help you become sensitive to your intuitive mind. Practice this meditation to move beyond fear and into intuition.

Meditation for Knowledge and Empowerment

Sit in a comfortable meditation posture. Keep your eyes open one-tenth and focus at the tip of your nose. Use your right thumb to block your right nostril and inhale through your left nostril. Cover your left nostril with your index finger and exhale through your right nostril. Continue breathing in this sequence while maintaining your eye focus. Practice for 3–31 minutes for 40 days.

Benefits This eye focus may be difficult to hold at first. Build this skill slowly. This eye focus locks your mind, creating a powerful energy that stimulates your optic nerve. The optic nerve stimulates the frontal lobe of your brain and your hypothalamus. Developing these two aspects of your brain results in a steady and penetrating personality. This strength is said to be re-

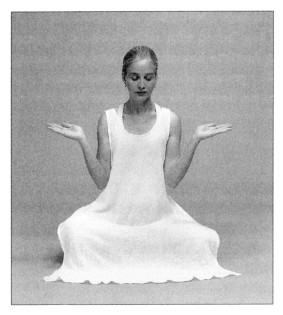

Meditation for Healing Yourself and Others

quired for the changes that are to come as we embrace the new millennium. This meditation will bring you the sensitivity to realize the truth of existence.

Meditation for Healing Yourself and Others

Sit in Easy Pose (cross-legged) or in a chair with your spine straight. Bend your elbows and place them by your sides, slightly in front of your ribs. Place your forearms straight up and bend your wrists away from you so that your flat palms are facing upward.

Close your eyes, hold the posture, and vibrate the following mantra aloud:

> *Ra Ma Da Sa—Sa Say So Hung*
>   (pronounced *rah mah dah sah—sah say soh hunng*)
> Sun, Moon, Earth, Infinity—Totality of Infinity, I am Thou.

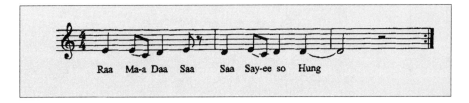

Continue chanting this mantra for 3–11 minutes. To end the meditation, inhale and suspend your breath briefly, and exhale. Repeat this breath sequence twice more, and relax.

Benefits The beauty of this affirming mantra is clear. You are not isolated from the divine energy of the universe. You are, in fact, one with that energy, always connected to bliss. You can direct the healing energy stimulated by the mantra toward yourself and/or others. The mantra is repeated aloud so that the tongue strikes the upper palate, which sends a positive signal to your brain and nervous system.

Moditation Sequence to Release the Past

Those who live in the past have no future. This meditation helps heal and release memories that negatively affect your ability to be in the present and enjoy your life. Sit in a comfortable meditation posture for the entire sequence.

1. Place your left hand in front of your chest with the palm facing to the right. Curl the fingers of your right hand and place your knuckles on the pads below the fingers of your left hand. Position your thumbs so they touch each other along their entire length (the bases of the palms of your hands should also touch). Hold this mudra in front of your chest, with your elbows bent. Form an O shape with your mouth. Breathe very slowly through your mouth with Long, Deep Breaths. Inhale and exhale through your mouth and feel the breath moving over your throat. Keep your mouth in the O shape throughout the breathing. Your breath will make a deep sound. Close your eyes and concentrate on the sound of your breath for 3 minutes. To end this part of the sequence, inhale and suspend your breath. Hold the breath as long as is comfortable, to a maximum of 1 minute. As you hold your breath, gather any memories, impressions, or experiences you would like to release. When you are ready, exhale and consciously release these images, feelings, and thoughts with your breath. Repeat this gathering and relcasing sequence twice more. Relax.

2. Bend your elbows and place them by your sides. Hold your palms by your shoulders, facing outward. On your right hand, touch your ring

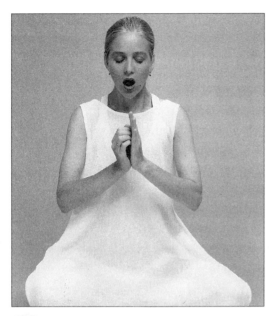

Meditation to Release the Past (1)

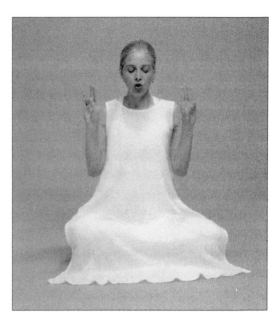

Meditation to Release the Past (2)

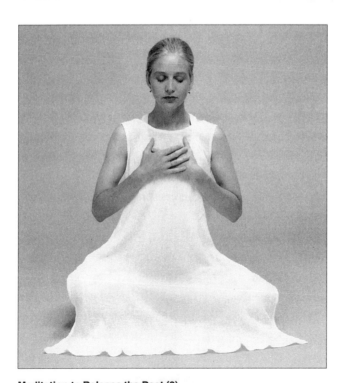

Meditation to Release the Past (3)

finger to your thumb. On your left hand, touch your little finger to your thumb. Hold this mudra. Form an O shape with your mouth. Begin a steady Cannon Breath through your mouth. This is a steady and strong Breath of Fire through the open mouth. Make sure you inhale and exhale equally and do not strain. Continue this breath for 3 minutes. To end, inhale through your nose, suspend your breath, and focus your closed eyes up toward the crown of your head. Then exhale and relax. Repeat the sequence of holding and focusing your eyes upward twice more. Relax.

3. Close your eyes. Place your hands over your chest—your heart center of compassion and love. Position them with your left hand under your right. Relax your breath. Concentrate on the light of your heart, your innocence, your peace, your beauty, and your bliss. Bless any thought that enters into your awareness. No matter what thought comes to you, bless it. Continue for 7 minutes. Inhale and suspend your breath briefly, then relax.

Benefits This sequence is an excellent example of using yoga as a healing therapy. You can start with less time for each exercise and build up to the times indicated as you continue your practice. This meditation will teach you how to encounter your own life, and then how to process and elevate your consciousness.

Meditation for Positive Thinking and Gratitude—Cup of Prayer

Sit in Easy Pose with a straight spine. Bring your hands together approximately 6 inches from the front of your chest. Cup your hands, with the edge of your right hand touching the edge of your left hand. Continue to hold the hand posture until you feel so relaxed that it seems your eyelashes are relaxing.

Benefits This meditation is one of the hardest to do! You simply sit and allow all the blessings of your life to fall into your hands. Merge with the light of those blessings and that divinity and feel them as a reality. As a result, you will feel a sense of gratitude and belonging.

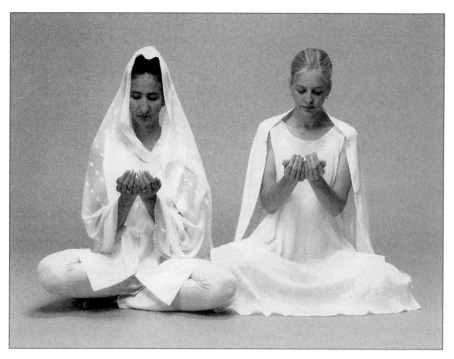

Cup of Prayer

"Sweet Dreams"—Exercises for Restful Sleep

To quote Shakespeare: "Sleep knits the raveled sleeve of care." In order to get enough sleep, you would need between 8 and 10 hours. Because of late-night television, computers, and lightbulbs, our brains are exposed to increasing amounts of light, and our biological clocks have extended closer to 26 hours.

Life-Nerve Stretch for Stress Relief and Restful Sleep

Sit with your spine erect and your legs stretched out in front of you. Keeping your legs close together, lean down from your hips and reach forward with your arms to grasp your toes. Relax your spine and allow your nose to come toward your knees and your elbows to bend and relax down toward the floor.

If the muscles of your lower and upper back and your hamstrings—the back of your legs—are tight, you may not be able to reach your toes. If this

A WOMAN'S BOOK OF YOGA

"I STILL CAN'T FALL ASLEEP!"

Here are some things you can do in order to get more and better sleep:

- Avoid late-night television and computer work.

- Avoid drinking caffeine after 4:00 P.M.

- Give yourself sufficient time and space to wind down in the evenings.

- Make your last meal light, and don't eat or drink late at night. Take a short walk after your meal to improve digestion.

- Take a calcium and magnesium supplement if needed. These minerals relax smooth muscle tissue, thus helping you to relax and sleep.

- Massage your body with scented oil.

- Drink a cup of warm milk or warm almond milk before bed.

- Steamed iceberg lettuce helps you sleep! Try some before bed. It has trace amounts of opiates and is very relaxing.

- If your legs are restless at night, you may be low in vitamin E and iron. Try 400 IU of each daily.

is the case, try the alternative: you can sit on a pillow, resting your hands on your shins or knees as you bend forward from your hips. Stretch your hamstrings by flexing your feet and pressing your heels away from you. Hold the posture for 30 seconds to 3 minutes with Long, Deep Breathing. To end, inhale and suspend your breath briefly. Exhale and relax.

Benefits This yoga pose can help you release stress. When you stretch the back of your legs, you are stretching your Life Nerve—the large nerves in your legs that connect with your parasympathetic nervous system that helps you regain harmony in stressful situations. During times of stress, practice

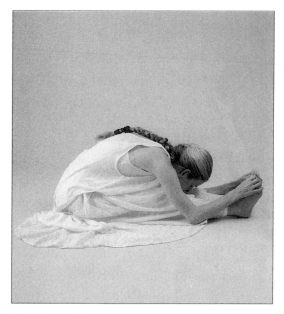

Life-Nerve Stretch

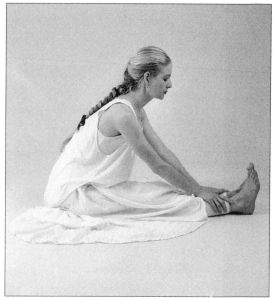

Life-Nerve Stretch Alternative

the Life-Nerve Stretch for 3 minutes every 3 hours, and before bed for a more restful sleep.

Cat Stretch for Release of Tension and Waking Up

Begin by lying on your back. Stretch your arms out straight from your shoulders. Bend your right knee up toward your chest, and place your right foot gently on top of your left knee. Keeping the knee bent, let your right leg fall over your left leg. Stretch your right arm along the floor until it is over your head. Gently turn your head to the right as you feel the stretch in your lower back. Come back to the center and repeat on the opposite side.

Benefits The Cat Stretch can be a gentle or deep-twisting stretch for your entire back, while providing a massage for your reproductive organs. Do not overstretch but strive to keep the bent knee and both shoulders on the floor. The Cat Stretch can be done slowly, holding the stretch for 30 seconds to a minute, or in a fluid motion as if you are rocking from side to side. Try the fluid motion Cat Stretch, stretching twenty-one times to each side in the morning while still in bed, to help keep your back healthy, release morning tension and stiffness, and give you a foundation of energy for the day.

Shoulder Stand for Digestion, Sleep, and Well-Being

Lie flat on a cushioned surface with your legs outstretched, your arms by your sides, and your palms facing downward to the floor. Take a few breaths. Bend your knees and bring them in toward your chest until your thighs press into your lower abdomen. Raise your hips off the floor, supporting your lower back with your hands, with elbows bent and your upper arms remaining on the floor. Only your head, upper back, shoulders, and upper arms should be touching the floor, with the weight held by your upper arms and shoulders. Avoid putting the weight of your torso on your neck. Position your hands toward the middle of your spine and stretch your legs up, straightening them. Gently point your toes toward the ceiling, keeping your legs together. Your elbows should not be placed any farther apart than your shoulders. Keep the knees bent if straightening your legs is difficult. To release the posture, slowly bend your knees toward your chest, and slowly relax

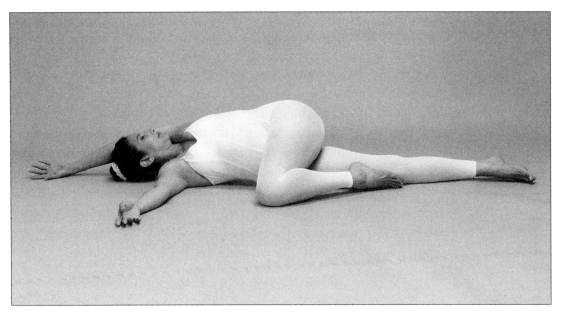

Cat Stretch

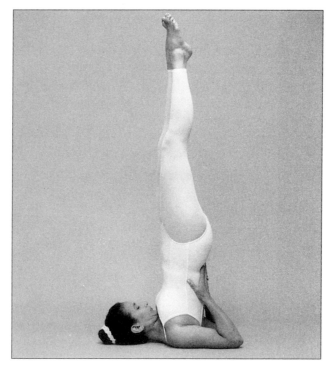

Shoulder Stand

your back onto the floor, supporting it with your hands on the way down. Relax.

Benefits The Shoulder Stand has long been considered an excellent daily posture for women. It allows healthy blood to circulate throughout the body, especially to the neck and chest. The thyroid and parathyroid glands in the neck are massaged and balanced as you hold the shoulder stand. The position of the neck, locked against the chest, can help eliminate chronic headaches. By inverting the body and thus reversing the gravitational pull on it, the digestive system receives a complete massage. This posture can, thus, help eliminate constipation and other digestive problems. The inversion also has a positive effect on the flow of spinal fluid, refreshing the body and brain, thereby creating a more restful physical and mental state in preparation for sleep.

Note: Do **not** do the Shoulder Stand if you have high blood pressure or an eye disease that is negatively affected by increased pressure. Seek the assistance of a certified yoga teacher for guidance.

Easy Breath Meditation to Help You Fall Asleep

Sit in a comfortable posture. Cover your right nostril with your right thumb and take Long, Deep Breaths through your left nostril only. Continue for 11 minutes, then relax. Wash your feet in cool water, and lie on your right side when you go to bed.

Modern Perspectives on Self-Healing

From both a medical and modern scientific perspective, yoga promotes self-healing by helping you fight the damaging effects of stress. Despite all the advances and marvelous innovations designed to make our lives simpler, better, and healthier, none of us is immune to stress. It affects us all, no matter what condition we find ourselves in: as members of a family with both partners working and no support from an extended family; as professionals changing jobs, selling a house, or retiring; as caretakers for ailing parents or young children; or simply as individuals living day to day with the uncertain future of our world. Stress is a toxin that can contribute to diseases of the heart, the intestinal tract, the immune system, and the mind. Stress can make diabetes harder to control and can even make it more difficult for some women to conceive. Stress may account for as many as two-thirds of office visits to physicians. These stress-related problems occur in part because stress leads to feelings of isolation. Many busy people find that there is no one available to nurture the nurturer and turn to their doctors for help.

Yoga is a universal antidote to stress that is available to everyone. Is it a miracle or a wonder cure? It is neither; the benefits of yoga are no more miraculous than good nutrition, exercise, and an enhanced awareness of your own mind and body. Yet yoga has much to offer to both the ill and the well. Yoga is not so much an alternative approach to health as it is a complementary one. To paraphrase the book *Mind Body Medicine* by Daniel Goleman and Joel Gurin, yoga is perfectly compatible with standard medical treatment and can be a powerful way of augmenting it, not challenging or replacing it.

Unfortunately, most of us have experienced firsthand the symptoms of stress—anxiety, trouble remembering, irritability, worry and restlessness, loss of interest in sex, and even depression. Stress affects our ability to eat and sleep in healthy ways and prevents us from fully relaxing. It can cause headaches, stomachaches, muscle tension, irregular elimination, and weight problems.

The relationship between stress and illness (and wellness, for that matter) has been observed and studied since the time of Hippocrates in the fourth century B.C. Yogis have also been aware of this relationship for centuries. However, it was not until the beginning of this century that Harvard physiologist Walter B. Cannon first described the *fight-or-flight response,* an internal process that helps the body adapt to a stress.

Faced with a dangerous situation, the body secretes powerful "stress hormones" called *catecholamines*, which prepare a person to either fight or run away. These hormones are produced by the inner portion of the adrenal glands, small glands located on top of each kidney, which is why the best-known catecholamine is called *adrenaline.* Other parts of the body also trigger the release of various chemicals and hormones, including *cortisol,* made in the outer shell of the adrenal glands. Cortisol is a potent hormone that over time suppresses the immune system, increases blood sugar, and creates feelings of sadness and anxiety.

The stresses that we experience today may still require the fight-or-flight response, but they are much more likely to come from psychological or interpersonal issues, such as family dynamics or the work environment. The end result of long-term production of potent stress hormones is chronic stress. Ultimately, chronic stress suppresses the immune system, and a comprised immune system makes us more susceptible to illness; causes the bones to lose calcium; increases muscle tension, which can lead to headaches; elevates blood pressure, which can lead to hypertension; and increases heart rate, which can lead to an arrhythmia, and more.

What has yoga got to do with all of this? A great deal. Much of how our bodies experience stress is controlled automatically by the *autonomic nervous system*, a part of the nervous system comprised of two divisions that balance each other. The *sympathetic nervous system* is responsible for the short-term physiologic changes mentioned above. Its counterpart, the *parasympathetic nervous system*, is primarily involved with relaxation and digestion. Yoga uses the parasympathetic nervous system to lower heart rate, blood pressure, and muscle tension, and these responses in turn help us recuperate from the negative effects of stress. Yoga also helps lower blood levels of cortisol.

HOW YOGA COMBATS STRESS

It's not the stress that makes us ill; it's how we react to stress that poses a hazard. While going to a yoga class may feel like one more destination in a busy day, once you're there you're able to tune out the world around you and tune in to your inner self, to slow down and focus, and to synchronize your mind and body. You learn to relax your musculoskeletal system, control your breathing, and increase parasympathetic activity, which dilates the blood vessels. With these skills you can relieve stress, oxygenate and nurture the cells of your body, and relax your harried soul.

These important changes enable us to take control of our selves and generate positive energy that refreshes and renews. By interrupting the cycle of wallowing in our own negative, repetitive thinking, yoga offers a means of combating overstimulation and regaining spirituality.

Recipes for Self-Healing

Jalapeño Milk

This recipe can help support your immune system when you feel a cold or flu coming on. It is also useful for depression. This food combination has strong healing properties. Be careful: The jalapeño peppers are hot! Start with just one-half to one pepper, and you will have a healing effect.

> ½ to a maximum of 5 jalapeño chili peppers
>
> 8 oz. milk
>
> A little honey (cuts down on heat of jalapeños)

Chop the jalapeños and blend them with the milk and honey. Sip slowly—this is hot!

Golden Milk

Golden milk is a delicious hot drink that helps keep your joints and bones healthy. The turmeric helps lubricate your spine and joints, and the calcium is excellent for your bones. This drink is also good before bed, as it is very calming. Women especially benefit from taking turmeric twice a week to support the hormonal system.

⅛ tsp. turmeric	2 tbsp. raw almond oil
¼ cup water	Honey to taste
8 oz. milk	

Boil the turmeric in water for about 8 minutes until it forms a thick paste. If too much water boils away, add a little more. Meanwhile, bring the milk to a boil with the almond oil. As soon as it boils, remove it from the heat. Combine the two mixtures and add honey to taste.

If you like, you can prepare a reserve supply of turmeric paste by boiling a larger quantity of turmeric and storing it in the refrigerator for up to 40 days.

For variety, try blending Golden Milk in the blender until frothy, and add a sprinkle of cinnamon.

Garlic Toast

Two cloves of garlic a day are considered a good preventive against illness. This is a tasty way to get your garlic for the day!

2–4 medium cloves garlic
2 slices whole-grain bread
Ghee (clarified butter)

Peel and thinly slice the garlic. Lightly toast the bread. Spread the bread with ghee. Top with garlic slices and broil for no more than 5 minutes (to maintain the potency of the garlic). Serve. Note: Garlic may be difficult for some people to digest.

Bananas

Eat one banana early in the morning and another at 4:00 P.M. with 1 tablespoon of raisins. This will help stabilize your blood sugar and minerals (especially magnesium).

Pears

Eat pears often to help heal iron deficiency in your blood. Pear juice is also said to get rid of fibroids.

Figs

Figs are an excellent food. They contain plenty of minerals, including calcium. The little seeds inside them cleanse your digestive tract and help elimination. Fresh figs are available occasionally; dried figs are available year-round. Try eating two figs each night before bed as an antidote to constipation.

Time-for-Sleep Tea

3 oz. valerian
2 oz. linden flowers
2 oz. kava kava
1 oz. catnip

Blend all the herbs together and store in a tightly closed container away from heat and light. Always keep to the proportions of the ingredients as indicated in the recipe. To make the tea, steep 1 teaspoon to 1 tablespoon of the herbal mixture in 1 cup of hot water for 20 minutes. Strain and sweeten, if you like.

Suggestions for Bringing the
Art of Self-Healing into Your Life

Read through the various self-healing meditations and exercises.

1. Tune in.

2. Practice a few gentle spinal exercises, such as the Spinal Flex or a rigorous yoga kriya of your choice.

3. Relax and meditate on the areas of your life that need healing. (You can also direct your meditations for healing toward anyone you know who needs help.)

4. Choose a meditation or healing technique and commit to practicing it for 40 days or more.

5. Commit yourself to developing your ability to perceive the lessons you need to learn from the challenges you face.

6. Compose and project a prayer for guidance and support in your efforts.

7. Long, Deep Breathing: Inhale as you mentally repeat *Sat* and exhale as you mentally repeat *Naam.* Continue for 3–11 minutes. Remember the meaning of the mantra—True Identity—as each breath links your personal identity with the universal truth. Every breath is bringing you the core alignment you need in order to keep up.

8. Project an intention of peace for yourself, those you know who need healing, and the world. Chant *Sat Naam.*

This process can set the foundation for your self-healing practice. It can be helpful to keep a journal or get support from health-care practitioners, family, or friends as you go through the process of healing.

QUESTIONS FOR FURTHER GROWTH

- What does "healing" mean to you?

- When life brings pain or disappointment, what is your most immediate response? How can you adjust your response so that you feel more empowered and relaxed, even during challenging times?

- What stops you from realizing your dreams, from standing up for yourself and your values? Choose a self-healing meditation, yoga exercise or yoga set, or lifestyle technique that addresses that issue.

- What areas of your life trigger your most negative sensations, physical or emotional? What steps can you take to heal yourself so that events or situations in your life do not negatively affect your physical, emotional, or spiritual well-being?

11 Natural Beauty

Woman is the molder. You are the molder of time, you are the molder of space and of man: The man of tomorrow, the child; the man of today, the husband; and the men of yesterday, the ancestors. The entire society, in theory and reality, is based on the spirit of woman.

—YOGI BHAJAN

Women's beauty is a big business. Even when styles and outward concepts of beauty change, society still defines beauty mostly by youth and outward appearance: by clothing, body shape, hairstyle, and hair color, to name just a few. Many of the products and services available to women, as well as the marketing and advertising that go along with them, promote a superficial concept of feminine beauty.

Real beauty has another definition. True beauty exists when the radiance of your soul permeates your physical appearance. By claiming your inborn divinity, and matching it with an outer projection and presence that represent your soul, you will experience true beauty. When your inner reality matches your outer projection, you will feel like you are "really you." You will feel a balanced relationship between your inner values and your actions in the world. Thus defined, *beauty* is the natural, balanced state of being and projecting yourself as the graceful, radiant woman you are.

In this chapter you will find suggestions for caring for your body that are based on this definition of beauty. If you try these suggestions in addition to committing yourself to a daily practice of yoga, exercise, and meditation, you will be caring for both your soul and your physical presence in the most positive way.

How the Yogini Views the Body

The yogis regard the body as a temple. Your physical body is an inherently beautiful vessel creation designed to carry your soul and enable you to follow your destiny in this world. Your body is a complete creation: There is nothing missing, and every part is important. The yogi sees the body as more than the sum of its parts and is careful to consider the possible effects on the body of any anticipated action. For instance, before making major physical changes, the yogi would make sure the change is for the best health of his or her entire being. In general, a yogi would not change the body just for fashion or vanity, because each part has a role in the whole creation. Nonetheless, any physical changes that enhance your health should be considered. The yogic philosophy is an attitude of respect for the body and respect for the divine intelligence that pervades the body.

The yogi sees the body as the divine instrument of experience. Through the body, you can experience pain, pleasure, and your Divine Self. All your senses, including your sexuality, are part of this instrument, and should be honored as important and respected aspects of your life. Your body is neither a commodity to be traded or sold, nor a source of sin to be subdued. The yogini sees herself as having a body, a mind, and a soul. Your totality includes a physical manifestation, a mental projection, and a divine presence that is beyond time and space. You are not your body, mind, or soul individually, but the web of life formed by the interaction of this trinity.

It may be unusual to seek such a multidimensional reality in a culture that has become increasingly superficial. How do you remind yourself of your true nature without getting sidetracked by advertising and the other pressures of the times? The yogini accomplishes this through a daily *sadhana* (discipline) of yoga, meditation, and relaxation. Practicing yoga helps you to maintain and sustain your true identity. This daily sadhana, combined with a sense of gratitude, will also help you maintain a more spiritual view of your body. The yogini consciously fights the tendency to view her body in media-driven terms and defines her beauty in spiritual terms.

The following yogic techniques can help you foster your inner beauty through the natural care of your body.

The Science of Hydrotherapy

Hydrotherapy is the science of healing with water. Water therapy is healing for women in many ways. Drinking fresh, clean water is healthy for your digestion and elimination, and for your skin. Swimming is excellent exercise for women. The motion of moving through the water can help heal frayed nerves, relieve fatigue, and lift your spirit. In addition to these activities, you can try the following forms of water therapy to enhance your natural beauty:

Cold Water Therapy

Healing through hydrotherapy includes taking cold showers, known in Sanskrit as *Ishnaan.* The thought of taking a cold shower may be strange to many women, but cold water is one of the secrets of remaining youthful. Hydrotherapy is considered a shield for good health—no exercise can match its effect. Asserts Yogi Bhajan: "In hydrotherapy . . . the water is a fatherly shield, *paanee pitaa,* and anybody who can produce this shield that conquers the coldness of the water can conquer death. . . . If I can conquer the chilliness of the water, I can take away the chilliness of my life."

Cold showers are not for washing your hair or cleaning your body. Rather, these showers benefit the health of your inner organs, your circulation, your skin, and your electromagnetic field (the energy you project). When the cold water hits you, your body responds with a change in circulation that is totally healing and cleansing. Your capillaries open and become flooded with an increased flow of blood. When they close again, returning to normal, the blood that has been released goes into your organs. Your heart, kidneys, lungs, and liver become flushed with the increased blood supply, which causes your glandular system to function more efficiently. Cold showers are an acquired taste. Don't worry about being too cold! Your blood flow will heat you up from the inside.

Overall, cold showers can help your glandular system remain balanced, increase your resistance to disease, strengthen your nervous system, and help your muscles release toxins. They also wake you up so you can meditate in the morning! Please note, however, that pregnant and menstruating women should avoid taking cold showers.

Cold showers may take a bit of courage, and that is part of the reason for them! If you give yourself a chance, cold showers are a fantastic addition to your natural regime and a powerful tool for managing your moods. Here are instructions for taking a therapeutic cold shower:

1. Massage your entire body with almond oil or olive oil. Almond oil has a subtle scent, so you can add a drop of lavender or sandalwood scent if you wish. You can also massage in the oil with a special pair of exfoliating gloves you can find at health food stores. The gloves boost the circulation of the massage.

2. Stand outside the shower and turn on the cold water. Step into the stream of water and let the water hit your skin while you vigorously massage your body. Chant (or yell!) the mantra of your choice as you enjoy the shock of the water. Do not allow the stream to directly hit your thighs. Step out of the stream of water after a few seconds and continue massaging yourself.

3. Step in and out of the stream of water four times, or until you begin to feel your body warming from the inside. You will begin to feel warm as the capillaries in your organs and skin are flooded with increased circulation.

4. When you have completed the cold water shower, massage and dry yourself with a clean cotton towel. You can also wrap yourself in a bath towel and let your body dry. After completing your cold shower, you can exercise, meditate, and relax for a complete and balanced healing yoga experience. Note: No cold showers during menstruation and pregnancy.

Headaches and Cold Water Therapy

If you have a headache, splash lots of cold water on your face. Put cold water on your ears and massage them. Your headache may disappear in just 2 seconds!

EFFECTS OF COLD WATER THERAPY

Here is how various parts of your body respond to experiencing cold water therapy:

- **Just below the lower lip**—creates clarity of mind

- **Between the eyebrows and the upper lip**—energizes you

- **Forehead**—makes you sleepy

- **Upper arms** (while you massage)—helps to heal your stomach

- **Elbows to about 2 inches above the wrist**—will help heal your digestive tract

- **Two inches above wrists to start of wrists**—hits the meridian points that are good for your heart

- **Wrist**—hits the meridian points that are good for your liver

- **Fingertips**—stimulates your brain

- **From the neck down your entire body**—improves cellular structure

- **From the chest and down to the genitals**—improves blood chemistry

- **Feet**—stimulates entire body

Computers and Cold Water Therapy

If you work with computers, take at least three breaks a day to wash your hands in cold water. Use a cold cloth to wash your face and put the cold cloth on your eyes and the back of your neck. This prevents the electromagnetic field of the computer from interfering with your nervous system. This advice has proved to be a lifesaver for many women who work long hours at a computer.

Immune System–Booster Hydrotherapy

Alternate cold/cool showers with warm showers. This can help stimulate your immune response and is recommended for arthritis and other auto-immune imbalances.

Natural Skin Care

Your skin is the largest organ in your body. All yogic practices will help keep your skin healthy. Moderate exercise—exercising until you sweat, but not so vigorously that you are out of breath—and hydrotherapy bring improved circulation to your skin and help detoxify your body. Your diet also affects your skin, so eating more natural, fresher foods can help the appearance and general health of your skin. Whenever possible, avoid processed foods, heavy fats, sugars, and foods that are hard to digest.

Severe and persistent skin problems may indicate liver imbalances and/ or unexpressed anger. Meditate and use other therapeutic techniques to help yourself heal from the inside out. Also try therapies that work on the skin itself. All these efforts—diet, skin care, and healing from within—can yield excellent results.

Natural Hair Care

Hair is an important part of your body's divine design. The hair on your head, legs, underarms, and other areas of your body plays an important part in your overall health. According to the philosophy of Kundalini Yoga, you should allow your body hair to grow to its natural length to keep your outer projection strong and your nervous system healthy.

There are many natural ways to take care of your hair without using harsh chemicals. Here are just a few suggestions you can try:

- Oil your hair with a healing mixture of almond oil and a few drops of sandalwood oil. A mixture of jojoba oil and rose oil is an especially healing mixture for curly hair.

- A traditional Indian remedy for preventing hair loss is to massage coconut oil into your scalp, then sit in the sun until your hair dries.

- Taking vitamins A, E, and C and lecithin supplements helps keep your hair in good health.

- Eating onions and olives can help balance your hormones and rejuvenate your hair.

- Comb your hair with a wooden comb to maintain the balance of your aura and electromagnetic field. Tie your hair up on your head during the day and braid it at night.

Massage

Your skin is constantly absorbing energy and releasing toxins. Daily self-massage is one simple way to keep it healthy and to develop a positive relationship with your body. You can give yourself a massage and take a cold shower, as explained in the section on hydrotherapy, or massage yourself without the shower at another convenient time. Use the highest-quality massage oil or creme possible, because any oil or creme you use is absorbed directly into your bloodstream through your skin. Food-grade almond oil, which is rich in minerals, is an excellent and cost-effective choice.

Use the following self-massage technique with a cold shower: Mix eight parts almond oil with one part sandalwood oil. Massage your entire body with this mixture. To massage your back, attach a roller to the wall and rub your back up and down on the roller to relieve tension in your spine, shoulders, and neck. Spend at least 15 minutes massaging your body. When you are finished, relax for 15 minutes and then take a cold shower. The oil on your body will enable you to withstand the cold water more easily. To finish your self-massage, dry yourself with a fresh towel for 10 minutes. This massage is a wonderful therapy for your body and mind.

Foot Health and Massage

Foot massage is a common practice for yoginis. Your hands, ears, and feet are microcosms of your whole body. Foot reflexology is the technique of massaging the foot to release tensions accumulated in other areas of the body. You can massage your foot with about 15–25 pounds of pressure in a circular motion. Foot massage is a powerful way to relax and to serve another, and is one of the most pleasurable activities the body affords! You can also walk barefoot on the earth, sand, and grass to help you feel grounded and relaxed.

For a relaxing bedtime routine, wash your feet in cold water and massage them before bed to soothe your nerves. If you have difficulty sleeping, and especially if you are staying up late, try massaging coconut oil into your feet at night. This techniques cools the body and mind and will help you fall asleep.

Natural Face Care

You can keep your face healthy-looking without makeup! Moderate exercise increases circulation to the face, which gives your skin a healthy glow. Too much exercise can dry the skin, and too little can deter the natural cleansing efforts of your skin, which results in blemishes or in an unhealthy paleness. Cold water therapy also keeps your skin bright. By trying some of these techniques, you may decide to cut back on makeup (if you wear it). As an experiment, try wearing less makeup or take a few days off from wearing foundations and other heavier applications. You may enjoy the results! The following natural treatments are healing and enjoyable.

Lime and Oatmeal Facial

Cleanse your face with a gentle cleaner. Apply the juice of one slice of lime by gently patting your face with the slice itself. The lime naturally exfoliates your skin, so your face may begin to tingle. Prepare some "oat milk" by mixing a small amount of fresh oatmeal with room-temperature water. Squeeze the oats with your fingers and mix until the water is milky white. Pat the "oat milk" onto your face. Relax for a few minutes with your feet up. If your skin is very dry, add some almond oil to the "oat milk" before you apply the mixture. After a few minutes, rinse and enjoy the results of the increased circulation to your face.

Relaxed and Beautiful Eyes

As a result of normal stresses and advancing age, your eyes can become puffy. At times you may also notice dark circles under your eyes, which may indicate a kidney imbalance (possibly caused by stress, dehydration, or lack of sleep). To take a break from the stresses of the day, place a peeled slice of cucumber over each closed eye as you relax with your feet up and breathe slowly. You also can moisten two black tea bags and place them over your eyes to reduce puffiness and relax the skin around your eyes.

Taking a bath is relaxing and healing. The clear water of a bath is a wonderful way to calm emotions, enjoy a bit of privacy, and reconnect with your body. When taking a bath, keep the water warm but not overly hot. Stay in the bath for a minimum of 30 minutes. This amount of time allows your reproductive organs to relax and adjust to the temperature change. Here are a few healing bath techniques and recipes. Enjoy!

Fighting with Father Neptune

This ancient Greek technique uses water to help release anger and frustration. Sit in a pool or in your bath with the water up to your navel. Begin splashing the water, pushing it with your hands with all your energy until you are tired. The combination of the healing water and the motion of your body will help release unexpressed or repressed anger. Afterward, relax in the water and enjoy the release!

Muscle Relaxation

Add generous amounts of both baking soda and Epsom salts to your warm bath. Together these ingredients help relax tired muscles, particularly when you are just beginning a yoga and exercise program. This combination can also help you detoxify from negative experiences and cleanse your body. Great recipe!

Yogurt Bath

Add a few cups of natural, plain, whole-milk yogurt to your bath. Homemade is best, but there are good organic brands you can buy in health food stores. Let the yogurt dissolve in the warm water and enjoy a bath that deeply softens your skin.

Aromatherapy

Add your favorite scents along with a natural oil to your bath. You can use premade formulas or create your own. In a saucer, combine 1 tablespoon of vegetable oil, such as coconut, jojoba, or almond (from your self-massage and hydrotherapy), with a maximum of 5 drops of essential scent, and add to your bath. Here are some scents and their positive benefits:

> Rose—feminine and relaxing
> Sandalwood—healing, aromatic, and romantic
> Lavender—relaxing
> Eucalyptus—stimulating, detoxifying (helps with respiration)
> Citrus—uplifting, stimulating, clarifying
> Bergamot—antidepressive, soothing

The use of essential oils and aromatherapy is a common and ancient practice. Your sense of smell is primal and acute; the aroma of your bath need not be overwhelming to be effective. The most effective way to use aromatherapy is by creating subtle scents.

Detoxifying Bath

Combine almond oil with a few drops of eucalyptus oil. Add baking soda and Epsom salts and soak for 30 minutes. Make sure you are covered with the water up to or above your navel point. After 30 minutes, let out the bath water. Step out of the tub and run a cold shower. Take a cold shower, using the hydrotherapy technique of stepping in and out of the water until your skin is red and the cold water no longer shocks you. Massage your skin dry and wrap yourself in a big towel. Drink a glass of room-temperature water, then relax for at least 20 minutes. This bath/shower combination is wonderful for your skin, your lungs, and your peace of mind.

Meditation for Blossoming of Your True Self

Sit in a comfortable meditative posture with a straight spine. Bring your hands in front of your throat center. Place the base of your palms together with the base of the right palm touching the base of the left. Keep your fingers spread apart and open. Your hands will be "cupped" as if they were forming a flower. Keep the base of the palms touching while you gently allow the fingertips and thumb tips to touch, as if closing the flower, and then open again as if the flower were blooming. Continue opening and closing the flower. Your eyes are closed.

Benefits Feel "I am infinity. I am the rose." Just feel as if you are blossoming, opening up. This simple meditation is relaxing to the feminine spirit. Your power is limitless. When you feel the limitations of worry or stress, take a moment to call on your inner resources, your true self and spirit. Call on your spirit and feel exalted.

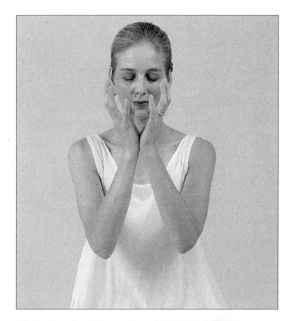

Meditation for Blossoming of Your True Self

YOGA AT HOME: NATURAL BEAUTY

Try the following suggestions to help you experience your own inner radiance and natural beauty.

1. Begin a daily *sadhana*—spiritual practice of yoga, meditation, and relaxation. Daily attention to body, mind, and spirit will help you develop a positive self-image.

2. Begin a daily practice of self-massage. Use high-quality massage oil and add scents that uplift your spirit. Self-massage is healthy for the body, relaxes the mind, and helps create acceptance for the natural changes every woman experiences. A sense of beauty begins with self-acceptance.

3. Either clothed or naked, sit in front of a mirror. Meditate on your own image. Then close your eyes and meditate on yourself as a perfect yogini, a goddess, relaxed and radiant. Open your eyes. Draw that image, write a poem about it, journal about the experience. How you think about your body and how you feel about your image can affect your actions. When you see yourself as an elevated soul, you can strengthen your resolve in achieving your dreams and goals and be content in the present moment.

4. Create time in your day to enjoy a special recipe bath or an invigorating cold shower followed by yoga exercises. Create space in your home to meditate, relax, and unwind. Dedicating time and space to personal care helps create a more positive relationship with your body and self-image.

5. Practice smiling. Say less and smile more. Your stress level will lower, and you will receive smiles from others. Smiling brings radiance and beauty.

- When you look in the mirror, what thoughts do you have about your body? Try not to waste time by overidentifying with the temporal physical appearance of the body. Your body will change as you age and journey through the cycles of life. Strive to connect with your spirit.

- When do you feel most beautiful? Notice if you are always looking for approval from others or comparing yourself to other women. Don't you feel most beautiful when you are relaxed and content within yourself?

And the Heart Lotus Blossoms Forth

Meditate for peace, tranquillity, happiness, joy, and bliss. Feel the energy of the Sun and Moon, the universe, all planets, all gods and goddesses, saints and sages, all good people, all kind people, all grateful people. They are all radiating the energy to you, and you are receiving peace. Fill yourself and take a part out of the universe and its nectar. Just meditate, and the petals of the flowers are being showered on you throughout the heavens by all the saints and sages, holy men, gods and goddesses. People of dignity and grace and virtue are showering blessings on you. We are blessed by Guru and gurus and by all those who came throughout time and gave the message of God. They are all radiating their light to you, and you are vibrating under that radiation.

Meditate and feel that the lotus of the heart is turning upward, the fragrance is spreading all around you, and you can smell a special smell of you, a fragrance of you. Feel the kindness of those great ones who attuned their lives to righteousness. Feel that they are in you, are around you, are by your side and that the radiance of their auras is filling up your mind. Focus your eyes at the tip of your nose and feel that the power of the universe is coming into you. Now radiate, and feel that all that radiance is making your life in this body transparent and that all opaqueness is vanishing. You are becoming transparent. Inhale deep, exhale, inhale deep, exhalc, inhale deep, exhale.

—Yogi Bhajan

Herb	Actions	Used for	Dosage	Concerns
Black cohosh (*Cimicifuga racemosa*)—root	Stimulates some estrogen activity by attaching to estrogen receptors; lowers luteinizing hormone (LH); may stimulate uterus	Menopausal symptoms (hot flashes, anxiety, and depression) best studied, but also for painful periods and premenstrual syndrome (PMS)	All dosages used 2–3 times daily. Tablets: 20 mg (standardized to 2.5% triterpene glycosides); extract (1:10): 0.3–2 ml, 60% alcohol	Mild gastrointestinal distress. High dosages can cause nausea, vomiting, dizziness, low pulse, and perspiration. Caution after 6 months' use.
Echinacea—flower head and leaf better studied than root	Antiviral, immune stimulant, antibacterial, antiinflammatory	Colds, chronic respiratory and lower urinary tract conditions, wounds, burns, eczema, psoriasis, canker sores, recurrent ear infections	All dosages used 3 times daily. Tea: 0.5–1 g; encapsulated freeze-dried plant: 325–600 mg; tincture (1:5): 2–4 ml; extract (1:1): 2–4 ml; solid extract to contain 3.5% echinacoside, 150–300 ml	Very few. Caution with autoimmune disease or medicines that suppress the immune system.
Chasteberry (*Vitex agnus castus*)	Increases progesterone by stimulating pituitary gland to make LH (luteinizing hormone). Lowers prolactin; mild sedative and antispasmodic	PMS symptoms, especially anxiety, depression, moodiness, and sleeplessness; some menopausal symptoms	Extract: 40 drops of liquid; tincture (1:5): 175 mg daily; tablets: 2 mg twice daily standardized to 0.5% Agnuside	Generally considered safe. Best avoided during pregnancy and lactation.

Herb	Actions	Used for	Dosage	Concerns
Dong quai (*Angelica sinensis*)—Do not confuse with *Angelica archangelica,* which has some of the same benefits as Dong quai but is more of a stimulant.	Phytoestrogen—binds estrogen receptor sites	PMS symptoms, regulating menstrual cycle, relieving a variety of menopausal symptoms, improving circulation and digestion	Tea: 1 tsp (2 g) of root slice, coarsely crumbled and steeped in ¼–1 cup boiling water in a well-covered container for 20 minutes; drink 1 cup 1–6 times a day; tincture: 10 drops to 1 tsp. diluted in 1 cup liquid, 1–6 times or more as needed each day, especially to assist in managing hot flashes. Also available as capsules	Avoid during pregnancy and during menstrual bleeding.
Garlic (*Allium sativum*)—clove	Lowers cholesterol; may reduce blood clots by prolonging bleeding and clotting times; fights certain bacteria and viruses; may reduce risk of stomach cancer	Stomach ailments, respiratory ailments, recurrent colds	Commonly standardized to 4–12 mg allicin daily. Available as 400–1,200 mg powder, 2–5 g fresh dried bulb; oil: 0.03–0.12 ml; tincture (1:5): 2–4 ml in 45% alcohol, 3 times daily	Odorless garlic usually much less effective. May cause flatulence, heartburn, nausea, vomiting, and unpleasant sensations in mouth; therapeutic dosages in pregnancy may increase risk of miscarriage.

Herb	Actions	Used for	Dosage	Concerns
Ginger (*Zingiber officinale*)—rhizome	Anti-inflammatory; improves circulation, reduces nausea; anti-spasmodic	Colic, gas and upset stomach; possibly motion sickness and morning sickness	0.5–2 g dried rhizome 2–3 times daily, or 1.5–3 ml extract 3 times daily. For nausea, 250 mg every 2–3 hours for up to 4 dosages; begin a few days before travel to prevent motion sickness	Do not use if gallstones are present. Higher dosages may cause miscarriage, but herbalists recommend 1–2 g dried root or prepared ginger daily for morning sickness. Excessive dosages should be discussed with medical provider if taking heart or diabetes medication
Ginkgo (*Ginkgo biloba*)—dried leaf extract: contains 22–27% flavone glycosides, 5–7% terpene lactones (ginkgolides A, B, C, and bilobalide), and no more than 5 ppm ginkgolic acids. Seeds also used.	Reduces blood clot formation; improves brain circulation and oxygen use by brain; improves painful walking due to poor circulation	Memory lapses, difficulty concentrating, depression, dizziness, tinnitus, and headache. Inhaling decoction of leaves used to treat asthma; seeds used for cough and congestion	Leaf extract: 80–240 mg daily; solid extract: 40 mg three times daily; fluid extract (1:1): 0.5 ml, 3 times daily	Generally considered safe. Gastrointestinal upset and headache reported. Seed can cause food poisoning. Extracts taken with blood thinners or aspirin may cause bleeding.

NATURAL REMEDIES FOR COMMON COMPLAINTS

Herb	Actions	Used for	Dosage	Concerns
Ginseng (*Panax ginseng*)—root: white ginseng is the peeled, sun-dried root; red ginseng is un-peeled, steamed, and dried. Root contains at least 1.5% ginseno-sides, calculated as ginsenoside Rg 1.	Lowers blood sugar; anti-depressant; anti-inflammatory; may improve mental function	Tonic for invigor-ating and fortify-ing when feeling weak or fatigued, and for improving ability to work and concentrate	For young and healthy: 0.5–1 g root daily as two divided dosages. Usually used for 15–20 days with a 2-week root free period. Best taken in the morning 2 hours before a meal, and in the evening at least 2 hours after a meal. For old and sick: 0.4–0.8 g root daily. Break not needed	Generally safe. Use with caution for cardiac pa-tients or patients with diabetes and those using MAO inhibitor medica-tions. If your energy level is normal, may cause uncomfort-able feelings of nervousness, insomnia, and hyperactivity.
Ginseng, siber-ian (*Eleuthero-coccus sentico-sus*)—dried root and rhizome	Stimulates im-mune system; lowers blood pressure; plays a role in digestive and glucose reg-ulation	Chronic inflam-mation, chronic fatigue syndrome, fibromyalgia, and chemotherapy. Used to revive strength and energy	2–3 g dried and powdered root and rhizome daily; solid ex-tracts stan-dardized at 300–400 mg eleutherosides B and E daily, or 8–10 ml 2–3 times daily. Usu-ally taken for 6–8 weeks with 1 week off and an-other 6–8 week course	Use with caution when taking stim-ulants, antipsy-chotics, or heart or blood pressure medications. Avoid if pregnant or breast-feeding. At higher dosages, insom-nia, anxiety, irritability, and palpitations can occur.

Herb	Actions	Used for	Dosage	Concerns
Licorice root (*Liquiritiae radix*)—un-peeled, dried roots and stolons of *Glycyrrhiza glabra*	Speeds healing of ulcers; helps break up respiratory secretions	Inflammation of the mucous membranes of the upper respiratory tract and stomach or duodenal ulcers	5–15 g of root, equivalent to 200–600 mg of glycyrrhizin	Can increase loss of potassium; therefore use with caution with diuretics and digitalis. Do not use more than 4–6 weeks without medical advice.
Soy (Isoflavones are the active ingredient.)	Natural plant estrogen (phytoestrogen)—inhibits growth of some cancer cells; slows down loss of calcium from bones	Menopausal symptoms, preventing osteoporosis, promoting heart health by improving elasticity of arteries; possible reduction of risk of breast, prostate, and colon cancers	Soy milk: 8 ozs. daily; tofu or soy nuts: ½ cup daily; soy protein: 40–50 g (usually two scoops) daily; capsules/ tablets: 25 mg isoflavones twice daily is preferable to one dose of 50 mg to maintain blood levels— SoyCare brand organic and GMO-free	Generally considered safe. May cause flatulence.

APPENDIX A:
NATURAL REMEDIES FOR COMMON COMPLAINTS

Herb	Actions	Used for	Dosage	Concerns
St. John's wort (*Hypericum perforatum*)—above-ground parts	Antibiotic; reduces inflammation; sedative and tranquilizing effect on brain	Treatment of mild depression. Used externally to treat wounds and burns	Tablets: 600–900 mg daily in divided dosages standardized to 0.2% hypericin or 2–4 g of total herb	May cause rash when skin is exposed to sunlight. May interact with antidepressant medications. Severe depression should be treated by medical professional.

Vitamin/Mineral	Possible Benefits	Dietary Sources	Concerns
Vitamin A (Beta-carotene) RDA Women: 4,000 IU Men: 5,000 IU	Essential for normal growth and for eye and skin health. Helps you see at night.	Carrots and dark green leafy vegetables, carrots, cantaloupe, and peaches as well as liver, eggs, milk, and butter. Beta-carotene is converted in the body to vitamin A.	Generally safe up to 10,000 IU daily. May be toxic above 50,000 IU. Doses above 20,000 IU daily during pregnancy may cause birth defects, but not everyone agrees that this is so. High dosages may increase the risk of lung cancer in smokers and osteoporosis. To minimize risk, look for supplements with beta-carotene as the major source of vitamin A.
Vitamin B$_6$ (Pyridoxine) RDA Adults to age 50: 1.3 mg Pregnant women: 2 mg Women over 50: 1.5 mg Men over 50: 1.7 mg	Helps the body process fats, proteins, and carbohydrates as well as build red blood cells and the immune system. May help prevent heart disease. Women in the United States typically consume less than the RDA.	Meats, liver, eggs, enriched grains, bananas, and peanut butter.	Dosages above 200 mg daily for several months could lead to numbness in the hands and feet and difficulty walking.
Vitamin B$_{12}$ (Cyanocobalamin) RDA Adults: 2.4 mcg Pregnant women: 2.6 mcg	Essential for normal cell development, especially blood cells, and for protein synthesis. Helps the body use fats and carbohydrates and helps the nervous system work properly.	Meat, fish, eggs, chicken, and dairy products.	Generally without risk in dosages up to 100 mcg. Individuals with abnormal intestinal absorption and strict vegetarians may become B$_{12}$ deficient during pregnancy, especially if they breast-feed.

APPENDIX B:
VITAMINS AND MINERALS FOR A HEALTHY DIET

Vitamin/Mineral	Possible Benefits	Dietary Sources	Concerns
Vitamin C RDA Adults: 60 mg	Antioxidant, protects cells from natural deterioration that results from aging. Also necessary to produce collagen, which makes up connective tissue.	Fresh fruits (especially citrus) and vegetables, green vegetables, tomatoes, and potatoes.	Dosages up to 1,000 mg are probably without risk. Higher dosages may cause diarrhea. Drying, salting, cooking (especially in copper pots), mincing of fresh vegetables, or mashing potatoes reduces the amount of vitamin C in foods. Pregnant women, smokers, and excessive alcohol consumers benefit from extra vitamin C.
Vitamin D RDA Adults to age 50: 200 IU Adults 51–70: 400 IU Adults over 70: 600–800 IU	Important regulator of the repair and formation of bone. Also controls calcium and phosphorous absorption from food.	Milk is the most important source. Exposure to at least 15 minutes of sunlight without a sunscreen also allows your body to form vitamin D. Older men and women and people living in areas where the days are short probably need a daily supplement of vitamin D.	Dosages up to 2,000 IU are safe. More than 5,000 IU daily can lead to irreversible kidney damage. People in nursing homes or those who do not get outside should consider supplementing with vitamin D.
Vitamin E RDA Adults: 30 IU	Antioxidant that protects cells from natural deterioration. Helps reduce the risk of heart disease and blood clots. Involved in making red blood cells.	Richest sources include salad dressing, cooking oils, and margarine, which together provide 30% of vitamin E in the American diet. Other sources include almonds, filberts, Brazil nuts, wheat germ oil, sunflower seeds, corn, asparagus, avocados, organ meats, butter, and eggs.	Studies have shown safety at dosages of 800 IU daily. Dosages of at least 100 IU daily appear to have a major potential to reduce the risk of heart attack.

Vitamin/Mineral	Possible Benefits	Dietary Sources	Concerns
Folic Acid RDA Adults: 400 mcg Pregnant women: up to 800 mcg	Helps reduce the risk of heart disease. Helps reduce women's risk of having a baby with a neurological birth defect. Needed for normal red blood cell development. May reduce risk of colon cancer and colon polyps.	Raw leafy green vegetables, peas, beans, citrus fruits, and fortified cereals.	The average American consumes only 200 mcg of folic acid daily, and cooking removes more than half of the folic acid in food. Pregnant women with a history of miscarriage or preeclampsia (a type of high blood pressure in pregnancy) or who take antiseizure medications may benefit from 800 mcg daily. More than 1,000 mcg daily may cause zinc loss or mask B_{12} deficiency.
Niacin (B_3) RDA Women: 14 mg Pregnant women: 18 mg Men: 16 mg	Helps process fat, produce blood sugar, and eliminate waste materials from tissue. Niacin also helps reduce blood cholesterol levels, which reduces the risk of heart disease.	Can be found in meats but also can be made in the body from the proteins found in eggs and milk. Often added to the flour in breads and pasta.	Safe up to 35 mg daily. Niacin supplements can cause itching, tingling, rashes, and occasionally a feeling of intense heat. Very high dosages of niacin can cause liver damage.

APPENDIX B:

VITAMINS AND MINERALS FOR A HEALTHY DIET

Vitamin/Mineral	Possible Benefits	Dietary Sources	Concerns
Iron RDA Women: 15 mg Pregnant women: 30 mg Men: 10 mg	Necessary for making red blood cells and hemoglobin.	Abundant in meats, eggs, lentils, nuts, leafy green vegetables, Cheddar cheese, and mussels.	Believed to be safe up to 75 mg daily. Needs reduced drastically in menopause. Absorption of iron may interfere with absorption of zinc, copper, and calcium. When taking supplements, add 15 mg of zinc and 2 mg of copper. Insufficient iron is a common cause of anemia, especially in children and women of reproductive ages, because of poor dietary intake and heavy menstrual flow and hemorrhage.
Zinc RDA Women: 12 mg Men: 15 mg	Helps red blood cells carry carbon dioxide to the lungs for disposal. Helps healing of wounds and keeping the senses alert. May help prevent colds and reduce risk of premature delivery toward the end of pregnancy.	Abundant in red meats, bread and other grain products, eggs, milk, sunflower seeds, soybeans, chicken, and seafood (especially oysters).	Safe up to 30 mg daily. Dosages of 2,000 mg daily can lead to vomiting.

Vitamin/Mineral	Possible Benefits	Dietary Sources	Concerns
Calcium RDA Children/young adults 1–10 yrs: 800–1,200 mg 11–24 yrs: 1,200– 1,500 mg Adult women Pregnant/lactating: 1,200–1,500 mg 25–49 yrs: 1,000 mg 50–64 yrs on estrogen: 1,000 mg 50–64 yrs not on estro- gen: 1,500 mg 65+ yrs: 1,500 mg Adult men 25–64 yrs: 1,000 mg 65+ yrs: 1,500 mg	Promotes healthy bones, prevents osteoporosis, and helps keep teeth strong. Also essential for muscle contraction and relaxation.	Milk, cheese, yogurt, leafy greens, broccoli, tofu, sardines (especially with bones), and salmon. If you don't eat much of these foods or are lac-tose intolerant, take a supplement.	Safe up to 2,500 mg daily. May reduce absorption of zinc and iron. Higher dos-ages can cause kidney stones, so be sure to drink at least 8 glasses of water daily. The mineral calcium is combined with one of sev-eral salts when taken as a supplement. These in-clude calcium carbonate, calcium citrate, and cal-cium phosphate. Calcium carbonate is the least ex-pensive but is less well absorbed. Calcium cit-rate and phosphate are absorbed more readily. Calcium phosphate has been shown to be better for building bones, as the process requires both these elements.
Chromium RDA Adults: 50–200 mcg	Helps convert blood sugar to energy. Helps insulin work effectively so may help prevent diabetes.	Healthful amounts found in peanuts, beer, cheese, broccoli, wheat germ, and liver.	Not recommended above 200 mcg daily.

APPENDIX C:
CALCIUM, CALORIE, AND FAT CONTENT OF COMMON FOODS

	Calcium (mg)	Calories	Fat (g)
Milk and Milk Beverages			
Milk, whole, 1 cup	291	150	8
Milk, low-fat (2%), 1 cup	297	120	5
Milk, low-fat (1%), 1 cup	300	100	1
Milk, skim, 1 cup	302	85	0
Chocolate milk (1%), 1 cup	287	160	1
Buttermilk, 1 cup	285	100	2
Cheeses			
American, 1 oz.	174	105	9
Cheddar, 1 oz.	204	115	9
Cottage, low-fat (1%), 1 cup	155	160	2
Mozzarella, part-skim, 1 oz.	207	80	5
Swiss, 1 oz.	272	105	8
Yogurt			
Plain, low-fat, 8 ozs.	415	145	3
Plain, nonfat, 8 ozs.	452	125	0
Fruit, low-fat, 8 ozs.	345	230	3
Coffee or vanilla, 8 ozs.	389	194	3
Desserts			
Ice milk, frozen, 1 cup	176	185	6
Ice milk, soft-serve, 1 cup	274	225	5
Ice cream (11% milkfat), 1 cup	176	270	14
Sherbet (2% fat), 1 cup	103	270	6
Other Sources of Calcium			
Almonds, 1/4 cup	94	210	19
Broccoli, cooked, 1/2 cup	47	25	0
Collard greens, cooked, 1/2 cup	179	30	0
Kale, cooked, 1/2 cup	90	20	0
Salmon, pink, canned, with liquid and bones, 3 ozs.	167	120	5
Sardines, canned in oil, with liquid and bones, 3 ozs.	371	175	9
Snap beans, cooked, 1/2 cup	31	18	0
Tofu, firm, raw, 1/4 block	166	118	7.1
Soybeans, dry-roasted, 1/2 cup	232	387	18.6

Hari Kaur Khalsa travels internationally, presenting workshops and seminars, and offering private consultations for women, men, and couples. To arrange for a workshop in your area, contact Hari via e-mail at ReachHari@aol.com, or at www.reachhari.com.

Hari also counsels women of all ages worldwide via telephone. Topics include relationships, sexuality, diet, yoga and meditation, and coping with the natural transitions of life.

Audiotapes are available on a variety of topics of interest to women. Students find these audiotapes invaluable as companions to the material in *A Woman's Book of Yoga*. The Illumined Women™ audiotape series includes:

> Kundalini Yoga for Women—A Beginners Series: Initiating the Feminine Energy
> Kundalini Yoga and Meditation for Perimenopause and Menopause—The Balancing Act
> Kundalini Yoga for Healthy Menstruation and Healing PMS
> Kundalini Yoga for Women—Food, Digestion, and Healing
> Kundalini Yoga for Women—Healing Past Traumas

Exciting video projects are currently being produced.

For more information on any of these resources, please write to me at the address below. I welcome your comments and questions and look forward to hearing from you.

> Hari Kaur Khalsa
> P.O. Box 44-1341
> West Somerville, MA 02144

3HO

The 3HO (Healthy Happy Holy Organization) is dedicated to spreading the teachings of Kundalini Yoga worldwide as taught by Yogi Bhajan. To contact 3HO or locate a Kundalini Yoga teacher in your area contact:

The International Kundalini Yoga Teachers Association
Rt. 2 Box 4, Shady Lane
Española, NM 87532
(505) 753-0423
Fax: (505) 753-5982
Web site: 3HO.org

Related Books

Yogi Bhajan, *The Teachings of Yogi Bhajan: The Power of the Spoken Word* (Arcline, 1977).
Shakta Kaur Khalsa, *Yoga for Women* (Dorling Kindersley, 2002).
Shakti Parwha Kaur Khalsa, *Kundalini Yoga: The Flow of Eternal Power* (Perigee, 1998).

For realated books and products contact Ancient Healing Ways at www.a-healing.com or (800) 359-2940.

Chapter 1

Begley, Sharon. "Religion and the brain." *Newsweek,* 7 May 2001, 50–58.

Chapter 3

Bera, T. K., Gore, M. M., and Oak, J. P. "Recovery from stress in two different postures and in Shavasana yogic relaxation posture." *Indian J. Physiol. Pharmacol.* 42(1998): 473–78.

Malathi, A., Damodaran, A., Shah, N., et al. "Effect of yogic practices on subjective well-being." *Indian J. Physiol. Pharmacol.* 44(2000): 202–6.

Raju, P. S., Kumar, K. A., Reddy, S. S., et al. "Effect of yoga on exercise tolerance in normal healthy volunteers." *Indian J. Physiol. Pharmacol.* 30(1986): 121–32.

Raju, P. S., Madhavi, S., Prasad, K. V., et al. "Comparison of effects of yoga & physical exercise in athletes." *Indian J. Med. Res.* 100(1994): 81–86.

Raju, P. S., Prasad, K. V., Venkata, R. Y., Murthy, K. J., and Reddy, M. V. "Influence of intensive yoga training in physiological changes in women: a case report." *J. Altern. Complement. Med.* 3(1997): 291–95.

Schell, F. J., Allolio, B., and Schonecke, O. W. "Physiological and psychological effects of Hatha-Yoga exercise in healthy women." *Int. J. Psychosom.* 41(1994): 46–52.

Telles, S., Nagarathna, R., Nagendra, H. R., and Desiraju, T. "Physiological changes in sports teachers following 3 months of training in yoga." *Indian J. Med. Sci.* 47(1993): 235–38.

Chapter 5

Seibel, M. M. *Infertility: A Comprehensive Text* (Norwalk, CT: Appleton & Lange, 1998).

Seibel, M. M., and Taymor, M. L. "Emotional aspects of infertility." *Fertil. Steril.* 37(1982): 137–45.

University of California at San Diego's Diagnostic Criteria for PMS.

Chapter 6

Sternberg, E. *The Balance Within* (New York: W. H. Freeman, 2000).

Chapter 7

Seibel, M. M., and McCarthy, J. A. "Infertility, pregnancy, and the emotions," in Daniel Goleman and Joel Gurin, eds., *Mind Body Medicine* (Yonkers, NY: Consumer Reports Books, 1993), 207–19.

Seibel, M. M., and Stephenson, J. *Journal Babies* (Mankato, MN: Apple Tree Press, 2002).